AF669603

Short Notes for Dental PG Entrance Examinations

Second Edition

Including Review for UG Students

Basic Sciences Volume 3

BDS III

Volumes in the Series

Short Notes for **Dental PG Entrance Examinations**

Second Edition

Basic Sciences

- **Volume 1** BDS I
- **Volume 2** BDS II
- **Volume 3** BDS III

Clinical Sciences

- **Volume 4** Operative Dentistry, Endodontics, Oral Surgery, Local Anaesthesia, Orthodontics, Pedodontics
- **Volume 5** Periodontics, Prosthodontics, Basic Radiology Self-Assessment Paper, Model Test Papers

Short Notes for Dental PG Entrance Examinations

Second Edition

Including Review for UG Students

Basic Sciences Volume 3

SANDEEP GOYAL MDS (Orthodontics)
Professor
Department of Orthodontics and Dentofacial Orthopedics
ITS College of Dental Sciences and Research
Murad Nagar, UP

Edited by
Sonia Goyal MDS (Oral and Maxillofacial Surgery)
Associate Professor, Department of Oral and Maxillofacial Surgery,
ITS College of Dental Sciences and Research, Murad Nagar, UP

CBS

CBS Publishers & Distributors Pvt Ltd

New Delhi • Bangalore • Pune • Cochin • Chennai

Second Edition

Short Notes for Dental PG Entrance Examinations

Volume 3

First Edition : 2006
Second Edition : 2010

ISBN : 978-81-239-1800-6

Published by Satish Kumar Jain and produced by Vinod K. Jain for
CBS Publishers & Distributors Pvt Ltd
4819/XI Prahlad Street, 24 Ansari Road, Daryaganj,
New Delhi 110 002, India.
Fax: 011-23243014 e-mail: cbspubs@vsnl.com; delhi@cbspd.com
Website: www.cbspd.com

Branches

- **Bangalore:** Seema House 2975, 17th Cross, K.R. Road, Banasankari 2nd Stage, Bangalore 560 070
  Fax: 080-26771680 e-mail: cbsbng@gmail.com
- **Pune:** Shaan Brahmha Complex, Basement, Appa Balwant Chowk,
  Budhwar Peth, next to Ratan Talkies, Pune 411 002
  Fax: 020-24464059 e-mail: pune@cbspd.com
- **Cochin:** 36/14 Kalluvilakam, Lissie Hospital Road, Cochin-682018, Kerala
  e-mail: cochin@cbspd.com
- **Chennai:** 20, West Park Road, Shenoy Nagar, Chennai 600030.
  email: chennai@cbspd.com

Printed at Somya Printers, Delhi-110053

dedicated
to
Ma Vaishno Devi,
my parents
and
my teachers

Acknowledgments

At the very outset, I bow my head to the Almighty God and my Guruji for all the grace showered on me to compile the second edition of the book. I am also thankful to my parents for their unforgettable sacrifices and choicest blessings.

I acknowledge the words of advice given to me by Dr Prof. Hari Parkash, Director General, ITS College of Dental Sciences and Research, Murad Nagar.

I place on record my deep gratitude towards my mentors and guides, my respected teachers during my postgraduation, Dr D N Kapoor, the then Professor and Head; Dr V P Sharma, Professor; Dr Pradeep Tandon, Professor, Department of Orthodontics and Dentofacial Orthopedics, Faculty of Dental Sciences, KGMC, Lucknow, for all their blessings, ideas and inspiration.

Prof P B Sood, Principal, ITS College of Dental Sciences and Research, Murad Nagar, has always been a constant source of insipiration and advice.

Dr Sanjay Tiwari, Professor and Head, Department of Endodontics, and Principal, GDC, PGIMS, Rohtak, for all his good wishes, the support, stimulating criticism and magnanimous help during my UG/PG days and afterwards.

My wife Dr Sonia Goyal MDS (oral and maxillofacial surgery), for her support, constant advice, contribution and editing the text, and all the pains she took during the compilation of the project.

Mr S K Jain and Mr Y N Arjuna of CBS Publishers & Distributors Pvt Ltd and their team of professionals for their best suggestions and help in getting this work published in the present form.

Last but not the least, I acknowledge all my family members and friends for their best wishes to boost my morale.

Sandeep Goyal MDS

Preface to the Second Edition

We thank all our readers for their overwhelming support and inputs for the first edition of our series **Short Notes for PG Dental Entrance Examinations**. However, with the increasing competition and increasing base of knowledge, a strong requirement for the improvement has been felt.

In the second edition, we have tried to incorporate a few new topics which will be helpful to postgraduate aspirants. We have now compiled the basic subjects and clinical subjects separately. This will help those undergraduate students also who aspire to compete for postgraduate entrance examination in the future. This edition will help and guide them to build their knowledge base from the very beginning of their dental career and will be helpful in their regular BDS examinations and also *viva voce* examinations.

We have included MCQs in this new edition for the side-by-side exercise and testing the skills and growth of their knowledge base. The book in the second edition has now been split into five volumes, considering the valuable additions made in the text as well new sections of MCQs which have been selectively added to strengthen the inherent appeal of this title amongst the potential readers. BASIC SCIENCES are covered in Vols 1–3 and CLINICAL SCIENCES in Vols 4 and 5.

We request our readers to continue sending their suggestions to us for future improvements for the benefit of their friends, juniors and other future dental surgeons.

In the end, we again emphasize that all the aspirants should synergize their knowledge by reading standard theory books to smoothly sail through the ocean of entrance examination, since our volumes may not be complete in every aspect.

Sandeep Goyal MDS
Sonia Goyal MDS
goyalsandeep2000@rediffmail.com
goyalsandeep2000@gmail.com

Preface to the First Edition

There has been a marked increase in competition in dental PG entrance examinations, which have become tougher in recent times. A proper guidance to the aspirants is, therefore, necessary for making their preparations.

The trend of today being MCQ-based, the aspirants just memorise the MCQs from the books available in the market without going into the depth of the statement, leading to errors during the examination. Also, a series of MCQs currently available in the market unfortunately contain 50 to 60% repetition of the questions, and the answers to many questions given in the answer key are also misleading and confusing for the students.

Most of the students do not want to undertake a detailed study of the subjects for their preparation and hence look for the easiest method to get through in the examinations which they consider to be present in the MCQ books.

In my view, MCQ books are for practice only. Your basic knowledge is tested through MCQs and they help to churn your mind, but you should not read them blindly thinking that they will be repeated in the examinations as such. The paper setters change the statements and options of the MCQs for better judgement of the student, therefore, only those students who have a strong basic knowledge can easily analyze and correlate the statement and the option. Also, for some of those students who read the textbooks and do not make notes but rather underline the text or write in the textbooks only, revision becomes very confusing and time-consuming.

This book has been compiled with an idea in mind to provide handy information in the form of a ready-reckoner to the aspirants. This volume covers eight important subjects, and other subjects will be included in the latter volume(s). The motive of compiling information in this manner is to bring important points of each topic together so that a student while reading the topics can revise all the key points immediately and at one stretch.

I have tried with the best possible efforts to tabulate and alphabetically arrange most of the important information so as to make it easy for the students to search for the required topic. The book speaks about the points to be stressed in the form of lists, like the most common terms, syndromes, synonyms, etc.

This book gives the students the guidelines and information about the topics most often asked in the examinations. However, they are advised to go for **further detailed reading from standard textbooks to supplement and reinforce their knowledge.**

I have attempted my best to include almost 80 to 90% of the important information on the covered subjects. However, the readers must study additionally and add their own points on the topics for their benefit.

No project can be completed and improved upon without **feedback**, constructive criticism and healthy suggestions. It is my humble request to all the readers and students to send me their suggestions and points/ topics to be added in further editions of the book, to make it more informative and useful for their younger friends and students. It is promised that these suggestions will be suitably incorporated in the future editions and all the contributors will be suitably acknowledged. My e–mail address is goyalsandeep2000@sify.com. Wishing you all the success in your examinations.

Sandeep Goyal MDS

Suggested Readings

Since we do not claim this book to be complete in all the respects, we advise the students to further supplement their information by going through other standard textbooks on particular topics. We are providing below a list of some books for reference for the students.

Author	Textbook on
1. Monheim's	Local anesthesia
2. Malamed's	Local anesthesia
3. Graber's	Orthodontics – an art or science
4. Profitt's	Orthodontics
5. Grossman's	Endodontics
6. Cohen's	Endodontics, i.e. pathways to the pulp
7. Ingle's	Endodontics
8. Gupta	Removable Partial Prosthodontics
9. Orban's	Dental and oral histology
10. Ten cate's	Oral histology
11. Shafer's	Oral pathology
12. Stone's	Oral pathology
13. Burkitt's	Oral medicine
14. Sikri	Dental Radiology, 4/e
15. Sikri	Conservative Dentistry
16. Goaz /White	Radiology
17. Singh	Embryology
18. Garg	Histology, 4/e

Standard books of MCQs which should be read definitely:

- ❑ Series of NDBs, i.e. national dental board papers, available upto L – series in I and II volumes.
- ❑ Rudman's
- ❑ Boucher's
- ❑ Steele's
- ❑ Gardiner's
- ❑ Cawson's
- ❑ Reed's Vols I & II
- ❑ Arco's Vols I & II

Besides these books, the students should always refer to the MCQ books available in the market for practice but they should not get confused.

Contents of Volume 3

Contents of Volumes 1 and 2

VOLUME 1 BDS I

VOLUME 2 BDS II

Abbreviations Used in the Book

AD	autosomal dominant
A.	artery
Ag/Ab/	antigen/antibody
Aka	also known as
Alv.	alveolar
Ant./post.	anterior/posterior
As	arsenic
Ass.	associated
B/W	between
Bact.	bacteria
BCC	basal cell ca.
C/E	clinical exam.
Ca.	carcinoma
Ch.	chronic/characteristics
Chr.	chromosomes
Cp.	compared
CT	connective tissue
Def.	deficiency
Dev.	develop/developmental
Dis	disease/distance as per the case
D/D	differential diagnosis
Enz.	enzyme
Epith.	epithelium/-al
ECA/ICA	external/internal carotid A
H/E	histology examination
IU	intrauterine
LAP	lymphadenopathy
LN	lymph nodes
LO	lateral oblique
M.	muscles
Mm	mucous membrane
MO/m.o.	malocclusion
Md/mand	mandibular
Memb.	membrane
MNGC	multinucleated giant cells
MNP/LNP	median/lateral nasal process

❑ Mo.	months
❑ Mx/max	maxillary
❑ n.m.	neuromuscular
❑ O/F	oral features
❑ Org./orgs.	organisms
❑ OTM	orthodontic tooth movement
❑ OMV	occipito-mental view
❑ OFD	object – film dis.
❑ PO	presence of
❑ PA	periapical/posteroanterior
❑ PNS	para nasal sinus
❑ Pt.	patient
❑ PDL	periodontal ligament
❑ R/G	radiograph
❑ R/L	radiolucent
❑ R/O	radiopaque
❑ REE	reduced enamel epith
❑ Reqd.	required
❑ SCC	squamous cell ca.
❑ SG	salivary gland
❑ S/S	signs and symptoms
❑ SMV	submento-vertex view
❑ Synd	syndrome
❑ TFD	target-film distance
❑ TOD	target – object dis.
❑ Vit.	vitamin

How to Prepare for the Entrance Examinations

This is my personal experience for PG entrance preparation and a time-tested method as many of my friends who have followed this method have been successful in the exams.

1. You have to believe in that hard work and luck go side by side.
2. Keep at least 6–8 months for preparation, which should be free from any sort of disturbance and forget about your surroundings.
3. Devote at least 8–10 hrs/day for the studies.
4. Divide your time and make a time bound schedule.
5. Pick important subjects first depending on the numbers of questions asked in the examinations. The subjects to be studied and stressed during entrance preparation are : general anatomy; dental materials; dental histology; pharmacology; oral pathology; fluorides; endodontics; periodontology; local anaesthesia; pedodontics; basics of all the clinical subjects.
6. Make your daily routine and diligently follow it.
7. Read MCQs two times from NDBs and any other standard book available on a particular subject. This will give you an idea about the style of MCQs and the part of the topic from which the question has been picked from the text, e.g. many MCQs are taken from the legends written below the figures in the book especially dental histology, periodontology, orthodontics.
8. Pick up a standard textbook which you have read during UG days. Read the topics and make notes separately and underline the important points. This will help you to strengthen your knowledge on that topic. Then take other subjects and follow the same pattern.
9. Read only relevant parts of the non-clinical subjects. Stress on anatomy, embryology, dental histology, pharmacology and physiology during the preparation.

10. All the topics and subjects should be covered in the time that at least two months are left for revision before the examination which you are preparing for.
11. When you have finished all the subjects, pick the MCQs books and read the 2–3 times. Any problem can be referred to your notes/textbooks.
12. Mark difficult MCQs in the book with different colors and read them carefully everytime.
13. 15 days before exams, read the notes on all the subjects, followed by one more revision of MCQs.
14. Discussion with your friends is a very important part of preparation. It gives an insight into the topics and more informations.
15. Take all the exams as far as possible; it tells you the trend; your standing and reshuffles your knowledge.

If you follow these rules, I can guarantee you 100% success in the examinations.

Syllabus

Given below is brief outline of the syllabus and topics the students should follow during preparation which should be supplemented by other topics for better knowledge.

Subjects	**Topics**	**Books advised**
Anatomy	♦ Head and neck — complete ♦ Brain — basics	Chaurasia's
Embryology	♦ Basics ♦ Pharyngeal arches ♦ Fetal circulation ♦ Fate of germ layers ♦ Development of oral cavity and face	I B Singh
Histology	♦ Basics ♦ Cell structure, cell division ♦ All glands and appendages, spleen, liver, etc. ♦ Skin, epithelium, A, V, N, M, CT	I B Singh
Dental materials	Complete	Skinners
Physiology	♦ Basics ♦ Blood, GIT, CVS, respiration, endocrinology	Chatterjee
Biochemistry	Basic concepts, enzymes, DNA/RNA, Krebs's cycle, HMP, etc. cycles carbohydrate/ lipid/ protein structure and metabolism, vitamins, minerals, energy requirements, etc.	Rama Rao, Harper's

Subjects	**Topics**	**Books advised**
Dental histology	Complete	Orbans
Dental anatomy	Basics, difference in morphology of molars, premolars, canines, mand lateral incisors, etc., occlusion, TMJ, alveolar bone	Wheeler's
Microbiology	Basics, sterilisation, structure of bacteria and virus, immunity, Ag–Ab reactions, *Strept.*, *Staph.*, *Clostridia*, *Mycobacterium*, HIV, Hepatitis virus	Ananthnarayan
Pathology	Basics only, neoplasia definitions, blood pathology (Do not waste much time on it.)	Robins
Pharmacology	Basic concepts, pharmacokinetics and dynamics, dental pharmacology, antibiotics, analgesics, LA/GA, sympathomimetic/lytic drugs, cholinergics/adrenergic, etc., briefly about CVS, CNS, antiepileptic, etc. Mechanism of action of all the drugs, MCQs	K D Tripathi
Oral pathology	Complete	Shafer's
Surgery/ medicine	Basics only, HT, TB, DM, infections, etc.	Any book
PCD	Fluorides, epidemiology, definitions, indices;	
Orthodontics	Basics, growth, ceph, diagnosis, appliances, wire properties, tissue reactions, forces, anchorage, tooth movements	Graber's, Proffit's

Subjects	Topics	Books advised
Local anesthesia	Complete	Monheim's, Malamed
Oral surgery	Basics; sterilisation, sutures, grafts, fascial infections, maxillary sinus, TMJ, salivary glands, fractures and x-rays	Kruger's, Killey's
Operative	Basics, cavity preparation, classification, cariolgy, instruments, cements and restorative materials, differences between cavity of silver, gold, porcelain, etc.	Sturdevant, Marzouk
Endodontics	Complete book	Grossman, Weine
Pedodontics	Complete book	Mcdonald's, Finn's
Periodontics	Complete book	Glickmann's
Radiography	Brief, basics	Any standard book
Prosthodontics	Basics of CD/impressions; materials, occlusions, jaw relations, implants, TMJ, movements, immediate dentures, etc.	Boucher's Fenn Winkler's
	Basics of FPD preparations, finish lines, crown preparations, principles, gingival retraction, impression, casting, etc.	Shillinburg Dykema
	Basics of RPD, DR, IR, connectors, classification of RPDs, diagnosis and Rx plan, surveyor, etc.	McCracken's Steward

BDS III

17

Oral Pathology and Medicine

SYNONYMS OF SYNDROMES

DEVELOPMENTAL ANOMALIES

Facial hemiatrophy	Parry-Romberg synd; Romberg syndrome	
Cheilitis granulomatosa	Miescher's synd	
Hereditary intestinal polyposis synd	Peutz-Jegher synd	
Labial and oral melanotic macule	Ephelis, focal melanosis	
Fordyce's granules	Fordyce's disease	
Focal epithelial hyperplasia	Heck's disease	
Fibromatosis gingivae	Elephantiasis gingivae	
Fissured tongue	Scrotal tongue	
Medial rhomboid glossitis	Central papillary atrophy of tongue	
Benign migratory glossitis	Geographic tongue, wandering rash of tongue; erythema migrans	
Hairy tongue		Hypertrophy of filiform papillae

Developmental Anomalies (*Contd.*)

Angiolymphoid hyperplasia with eosinophils	Kimura's disease; eosinophilic lymphoid granuloma	
Lymphoepithelial cyst	Branchial cyst	
Developmental lingual mandibular salivary gland depression	Static bone/cyst cavity, lingual mandibular bone cavity; STAFNE'S cyst	
Dens in dente	Dens invaginatus; pregnant tooth; dilated composite odontome	
Dens evaginatus	Leong's premolars; occlusal enamel pearl	Tratman's odontome
Amelogenesis imperfecta	Hereditary enamel dysplasia, hereditary brown opalescent teeth	
Dentinogenesis imperfecta	Hereditary opalescent dentin	
Dentin dysplasia	Rootless teeth	
Regional odontodysplasia	Ghost teeth; odontogenic imperfecta	
Ankylosed Submerged teeth deciduous tooth		
Median anterior maxillary cyst	Nasopalatine duct cyst; incisive canal cyst	Most common develop-mental cyst
Nasoalveolar cyst	Nasolabial cyst; Klestadt's cyst	

Developmental Anomalies (*Contd.*)

Palatal cyst of neonate	Epstein's pearls; Bohn's nodules	
Benign cervical lymphoepithelial cyst	Branchial cleft cyst; lateral cervical cyst	Close to anterior border of SCM m.

TUMORS OF ORAL CAVITY

Keratoacanthoma	Self healing carcinoma; verrucoma; molluscum sebaceum	
Pigmented cellular nevus	Pigmented mole; benign melanocytic nevus	
Erythroplakia	Erythroplasia of Queyrat	
Basal cell ca.	Rodent ulcer	
Epidermoid ca.	Squamous cell ca.	
Spindle cell ca.	Lane tumor; pseudo-sarcoma	
Adenoid SCC	Adenoacanthoma	
Peripheral ossifying fibroma	Peripheral odontogenic/ cementifying fibroma; calcifying or ossifying epulis	
Central ossifying fibroma of bone	Central fibroosteoma	
Peripheral giant cell granuloma	Osteoclastoma; giant cell epulis; PGC reparative granuloma	

Tumors of Oral Cavity (*Contd.*)

Verruciform xanthoma	Histiocytosis–Y	
Hemangioma	Vascular nevus	
Encephalo–trigeminal angiomatosis	Sturge-Weber disease	
Benign chondroblastoma	Codman's tumor; epiphyseal chondromatous GC tumor	
Benign osteoblastoma	Giant osteoid osteoma	
Kaposi's sarcoma	Multiple idiopathic hemorrhagic sarcoma of Kaposi; angio-reticuloendothelioma	
Ewing's sarcoma	Round cell sarcoma; endothelial myeloma	
Osteosarcoma	Osteogenic sarcoma	
African jaw lymphoma	Burkitt's lymphoma	EBV; children; B–cells
Multiple myeloma	Plasma cell myeloma; plasmacytoma	Punched out lesions in R/G; Bence–Jones proteins
Traumatic neuroma	Amputation neuroma	From perineurium
MEN - II synd	Sipple's synd	
Neurofibroma	Von–Recklinghausen's dis of skin; neurofibromatosis	
Neurolemmoma	Schwannoma; perineural fibroblastoma	

TUMORS OF SALIVARY GLANDS

Pleomorphic adenoma	Mixed tumor; enclavoma	
Papillary cystadenoma lymphomatosum	Warthin's tumor; adenolymphoma	
Oxyphilic adenoma	Oncocytoma; acidophillic adenoma	
Benign lymphoepithelial lesion	Mikulicz's dis	
Sjogren's synd	Sicca synd; Gougerat – Sjogren synd	
Adenoid cystic ca.	Cylindroma	
Acinic cell ca.	Adenocarcinoma	Lymphoid elements
Mucoepidermoid ca.		Most common malig salivary gland tumor in children
Donath–Seifert tumor	Clear cell ca. as epithelial–myoepithelial ca. of intercalated duct origin	

CYSTS AND TUMORS OF ODONTOGENIC ORIGIN

Apical periodontal cyst	Radicular; periapical; dental root end cyst, etc.	
Dental lamina cyst of newborn	Epstein's pearls; Bohn's nodules	Along midpalatal raphe, at the junction of palates

Cysts and Tumors of Odontogenic Origin (*Contd.*)

OKC		Highest recurrence
Jaw cyst–basal cell nevus–bifid rib synd	Gorlin–Goltz synd; hereditary cutaneo-mand polyoncosis	OKC; BCC; eye; CNS gonads affected
Calcifying odontogenic cyst	Gorlin cyst; CEOC	Ghost cells
Enameloma	Enamel drop; enamel pearl	
Ameloblastoma	Adamantinoma; multilocular cyst	Honey comb/soap bubble appearance on R/G; highly radioresistant
Calcifying epithelial odontogenic tumor	Pindborg tumor	Honey comb pattern; driven snow appearance; homogenous eosinophilic substance; calcifications in the form of Liesegang rings
Adenomatoid odontogenic tumor	Adenoameloblastoma	Duct like structures; resembles dentigerous cyst but extends beyond CEJ
Peripheral odontogenic fibroma	Peripheral ossifying fibroma; calcifying fibrous epulis	Arises b/w teeth; cuffing calcifications.

Cysts and Tumors of Odontogenic Origin (*Contd.*)

Periapical cemental dysplasia	Cementoma, cementifying fibroma, cementoblastoma	Associated with vital teeth; seen in 3 stages; occur in and near the PDL around apex
Benign cementoblastoma	True cementoma	With vital teeth; mostly mandibular 1st molar

REGRESSIVE ALTERATIONS OF TEETH

Dentinal sclerosis	Transparent dentin	
Secondary dentin	Irregular dentin	
Internal resorption	Pink tooth of Mummery; odontoclastoma; internal granuloma;	
Hypercementosis	Cementum hyperplasia	

BACTERIAL, VIRAL INFECTIONS

Scarlet fever	Scarlatina	
Sarcoidosis	Boeck's sarcoid; Besnier-Boeck – Schaumann dis	Kveim–Siltzbach test
Uveoparotid fever	Hereford's synd;	7th N paralysis; bilateral enlargement of parotid; eye's uveitis

Bacterial, Viral Infections (*Contd.*)

Leprosy	Hansen's dis	
Actinomycosis	Ray fungus	Sulfur granules; A. israelii
Botrymycosis	Bacterial actinophytosis; actinobacillosis	
Tetanus	Lock jaw	*Clostridium tetani*; risus sardonicus; ophisthotonus; blocking of spinal inhibition
Syphilis	Lues	Treponema pallidum; Hutchinson's triad; chancre → mucous patch → gumma
Granuloma inguinale	Donovanosis	Donovan bodies; by calymma-tobacterium granulomatis
Rhinoscleroma	Scleroma	Hebra nose
Noma	Cancrum oris; gangrenous stomatitis	
ANUG	Vincent's infection; trench mouth; fusospirochetal gingivitis;	Borrelia vincenti; punched out appearance of I/D papillae
Crohn's dis	Inflammatory gingival hyperplasia with regional enteritis	

Bacterial, Viral Infections (*Contd.*)

Papillon Lefevre synd	Juvenile/precocious perodontosis with palmar–planter hyperkeratosis	

VIRAL INFECTIONS

Herpes simplex	Cold sores; fever blisters; acute herpetic gingivostomatitis	HSV; balooning degeneration Lipschutz bodies; virus reside in regional ganglia; lesions develop on tightly bound mucosa
Herpetic whitlow	Recurrent herpes of hands and fingers	
Recurrent aphthous stomatitis	Aphthous ulcers; canker sores	
Sutton's dis or Mikulicz's scarring	Periadenitis mucosa necrotica recurrens	
Behcet's synd Reiter's synd		By PPLO Tetrad = urethritis; arthritis; conjunctivitis; mucocutaneous lesions; PPLO
Herpangina	Aphthous pharyngitis	
Measles	Rubeola; Morbilli	
Rubella	German measles	
Small pox	Variola	

VIRAL INFECTIONS (*Contd.*)

Chicken pox	Varicella	
Herpes zoster	Shingles; zona	
Mumps	Epidemic parotitis	

FUNGAL DISEASES

North American blastomycosis	Gilchrist's dis	
South American blastomycosis	Lutz's dis, paracoccidioido-mycosis	
Histopl smosis	Darling's dis	By birds excreta
Coccidioidomycosis	Valley fever; San Joaquin valley fever	
Cryptococcosis	Torulosis; European blastomycosis	
Candidiasis	Thrush; moniliasis; candidiasis	
Phycomycosis	Mucormycosis	Diabetes mellitus

PULP DISEASES

Chronic hyperplastic pulpitis	Pulp polyp	
PA granuloma	Apical peridontitis	
Chronic focal sclerosing osteomyelitis	Condensing osteitis	

Pulp Diseases (*Contd.*)

Chronic osteomyelitis with proliferative periostitis	Garre's chronic non-suppurative sclerosing osteitis; periostitis ossificans	
Cellulitis	Phlegmon	
Bruxism	Night grinding; bruxomania	
Traumatic cyst	Solitary bone cyst; unicameral bone cyst; simple bone cyst; idiopathic bone cavity; hemorrhagic cyst	
Traumatic ulcers	Decubitus ulcer/sore spots	
Inflammatory fibrous hyperplasia	Epulis fissuratum; denture injury tumor	
Inflammatory papillary hyperplasia	Palatal pappillomatosis	
Perleche	Angular cheilitis/ cheilosis	
Mucous retention cyst	Mucocele	
Acrodynia	Pink disease; Swift's dis.	Hg toxicity reaction
Argyria		Ag toxicity
Angioneurotic oedema	Quincke's edema; giant urticaria	
Drug allergy	Stomatitis/dermatitis medicamentosa	

Pulp Diseases (*Contd.*)

Contact stomatitis/ dermatitis	Stomatitis/dermatitis venenata	
Dry socket	Localised acute alveolar osteomyelitis; Alveolar osteitis; alevolitis sicca dolorosa;	

METABOLIC DISTURBANCES

Hurler's synd	Mucopolysac-charidosis 1; MPS 1 H; gargoylism	Typical spacing b/w teeth; p.o. gargoyle cells
Hand–Schuller–Christian dis (histiocytosis X dis)	Multifocal eosinophillic granuloma	Triad = diabetes insipidus + punched out bone lesions + exophthalmos; Foam cells
Gaucher's dis; is a lipid reticuloendo-theliosis		Gaucher's cells have "crumpled silk" cytoplasm
Osteomalacia	Adult rickets	
Vit D resistant	Familial	
rickets	hypophosphatemia, phosphate diabetes; refractory rickets	
Renal rickets	Renal osteodystrophy	
Hypophosphatasia	Hypophosphatasemia	Deficiency in enz. Alk Pase; **no cementum**; so no functional PDL

Metabolic Disturbances (*Contd.*)

Secondary hyperparathyroidism	Von–Recklinghausen's dis of bones	Brown tumors
Chronic insufficiency of adrenal cortex	Addision's dis	
Progeria	Hutchinson – Gilford synd	

DISEASES OF BONES

Osteogenesis imperfecta	Brittle bones; Lobstein's dis	Vrolik's type; Lobstein's type; blue sclera; DI
Infantile cortical hyperostosis	Caffey's dis; Caffey–Silverman synd	Arises during first 3 months of life; unilateral mandibular enlargement; increased Alk. Pase levels
Cleidocranial dysplasia	Marie and Sainton's dis;	Sunken saggital suture; prolonged retention of deciduous teeth; absence of cementum on erupted teeth; many supernumerary teeth
Craniofacial dysostosis	Crouzon dis/synd	

Diseases of Bones (*Contd.*)

Mandibulofacial dysostosis	Treacher Collins synd; Franceschetti synd	Eye; ear; face; hair; skeletal tissues affected
Pierre–Robin synd	Robin anomalad	Cleft palate + micrognathia + glossoptosis; bird facies; hypoplastic mandible
Marfan synd	Arachnodactyly	Deep palate; spidery fingers; flat foot; bifid uvula; multiple cysts, C/I orthodontic Rx
Down synd	Trisomy 21 synd; mongolism	Class III; open mouth; large tongue; caries free due to excessive salivation; deficient maxilla
Osteopetrosis	Marble bone dis; Albers–Schonberg dis; osteosclerosis	Dense sclerotic bone; roots of teeth nearly invisible; osteomyelitis develops very easily; normal serum alk. Pase
Achondroplasia		Class III due to deficient maxilla;
Osteitis deformans	Paget's dis of bone	Mosaic bone pattern; cotton wool appearance

Diseases of Bones (*Contd.*)

Generalised cortical hyperostosis	Van Buchem dis; endosteal hyperostosis	
Massive osteolysis	Vanishing bone; disappearing bone; phantom bone; Gorham synd;	
Jaffe's type fibrous dysplasia		Involves a number of bones; café au lait spots;
Albright's synd	Fibrous dysplasia with endocrine disturbances	
Cherubism	Familial fibrous dysplasia of the jaws;	A giant cell lesion; bilateral; absence of many permanent teeth and lack of eruption
Osteoarthritis	Degenerative joint dis	
MPDS	TMJ PDS	

DISEASES OF BLOOD

Pernicious anaemia	Addison's anaemia, Biermer's anaemia	- Deficiency of extrinsic factor, i.e. vit B_{12}; malabsorption of intrinsic factor; - TRIAD= generalised weakness, sore tongue; numbness of limbs;

Diseases of Blood (*Contd.*)

		- HUNTER / Moeller's glossitis - Howell Jolley bodies
Sprue	Celiac disease; idiopathic steatorrhea	Glossitis due to atrophy of filiform papillae; GLUTEN –free diet is useful in Rx.
Gee-Herter's dis	Celiac dis in CHILDREN	
Thalassemia Contains Hb-F; Increased serum bilirubin, osteoporosis	Cooley's anemia; medi-terranean dis; erythroblastic anemia	Diminished synthesis of α- & β - chains of Hb A; RBCs appear as TARGET CELLS; **safety – pin cells, Crew cut / hair on end** appearance on R/G; **salt and pepper effect** of trabeculae
Plummer-Vinson synd	Iron deficiency anemia	Development of carcinoma in upper GIT; decreased HCl in stomach
Polycythemia vera	Polycythemia rubra vera; Vaquez's dis; Osler's dis	Cyanosis due to p.o reduced Hb > 5 gm %. Splenomegaly

Diseases of Blood (*Contd.*)

Agranulocytosis	Granulocytopenia;	No apparent inflammatory infiltration around lesions
Cyclic neutropenia	Cyclic agranulocytic angina	Cycle repeats every 3 weeks
Infectious mononucleosis	Glandular fever; kissing dis	EBV; +ve Paul-Bunnel test; increased heterophil Ab titer; cervical LAP occurs first
Aldrich syndrome	Wiskott-Aldrich synd	Patient is not able to form Abs vs polysaccharide containing organisms
Familial thrombasthenia	Glanzmann thrombasthenia	
Thrombocytopathic purpura	Thrombocytopathia	Portsmouth synd; storage pool dis
Hemophilia	Bleeder's dis; Hapsburgs dis; the dis of KINGS	
Von Willebrand's dis	Pseudohemophilia; vascular hemophilia/ purpura	By decrease in all 3 components of factor 8; only BT is prolonged
Macroglobulinemia	Macroglobulinemia of Waldenstrom	Bence Jones proteins may be +nt.

BLOOD CLOTTING FACTORS: (mnemonic = *face per tere chunri laal **n**ahin sajti; **a**isi chunri se **p**areshan **h**ai face.*)

1. ***F***ibrinogen
2. ***P***rothrombin
3. ***T***hromboplastin
4. ***C***alcium
5. ***L***abile factor/proaccelerin
6. ***N***o longer used
7. ***S***table factor/prothrombin conversion accelerator
8. ***A***ntihemophilic globulin
9. ***P***lasma thromboplastin component/Christmas factor
10. ***S***tuart factor
11. ***P***lasma thromboplastin antecedent
12. ***H***ageman factor
13. ***F***ibrin stabilising factor

DISEASES OF SKIN

Hereditary hypohydrotic ectodermal dysplasia	Hereditary anhydrotic ectodermal dysplasia	
Chondroectodermal dysplasia	Ellis-van Creveld synd	
Erythema multiforme	Stevens-Johnson synd	Target/bull/eye lesions; Skin, oral cavity, genitals and eyes are involved
Mucocutaneous lymph node synd	Kawasaki dis	
Keratosis follicularis	Darier's dis, Darier – White's dis	

Diseases of Skin (*Contd.*)

Warty dyskeratoma	Isolated Darier's dis	
Incontinentia pigmenti	Bloch-Sulzberger synd	
White sponge nevus	Cannon's dis; oral epithelial nevus;	
Familial benign chronic pemphigus	Hailey-Hailey dis	
Cicatricial pemphigoid	Ocular pemphigus; benign mucous memb pemphigoid	+ve fluorescence at basement zone; tissue bound basement memb Abs
Epidermolysis bullosa simplex, localized form	Weber-Cockayne synd	
Junctional epidermolysis bullosa	Herlitz's dis	
Dermatitis herpetiformis	Duhring-Brocq dis	
Systemic sclerosis	Scleroderma; Hidebound dis	Raynaud's phenomenon is always +nt; CREST Synd; mask like skin; ivory white waxy skin; extreme widening of PDL
Ehlers-Danlos synd	Cutis hyperelastica	Rubber man; suturing not possible; lack of normal scalloping of DEJ

Diseases of Skin (*Contd.*)

Focal dermal hypoplasia synd	Goltz-Gorlin synd	Focal absence of dermis; a mesoectodermal dysplasia
Solar elastosis	Senile/actinic elastosis.	

DISEASES OF NERVES AND TMJ

Trigeminal	Tic douloureux; Fothergill's dis;	Trigger zones;
Trotter's synd neuralgia	Pain as trigeminal neuralgia and mid ear deafness due to NASOPHARYN-GEAL Ca.	
Paratrigeminal synd Sphenopalaine neuralgia	Raeder's synd Horton's synd; Sluder's headache; lower half headache; vidian nerve neuralgia; cluster headache	Alarm clock headache;
Orolingual paresthesia	Glossodynia; glossopyrosis	
Auriculotemporal synd	Frey's synd; gustatory sweating	
Bell's palsy	Facial nerve paralysis	
Melkersson-	Bell's palsy + facial	
Rosenthal synd	edema + cheilitis granulomatosa + fissure tongue	

Diseases of Nerves and TMJ (*Contd.*)

Horner's synd	Sympathetic ophthalmoplegia	Triad = miosis + ptosis + anhidrosis
Jaw winking synd	Marcus-Gunn phenomenon; pterygoid – levator synkinesis	
Marin-Amat synd	Inverted Marcus – Gunn phenomenon	
Congenital myotonia	Thomsen's dis	
Mobius synd	Congenital facial diplegia	

TYPICAL RADIOGRAPHIC APPEARANCE OF DIFFERENT CYSTS

Cysts	Appearance	
Radicular	Unilocular radiolucency at apex of tooth	
Residual	Unilocular periapical radiolucency at an extraction site	
Dentigerous	Radiolucency around an impacted tooth attached to its CEJ	
OKC	Multilocular radiolucency at angle of mandible	
Eruption	Unilocular radiolucency around an erupting tooth	
CEOC	Well-defined unilocular radiolucency mostly between lower anteriors and having small calcific masses	

Typical Radiographic Appearance of Different Cysts (*Contd.*)

Cysts	Appearance	
Static bone cavity	Ovoid radiolucency below mandibular canal	
Traumatic bone cyst	Scalloped radiolucency along the roots above mandibular canal	
Incisive canal/ nasopalatine	Heart shaped radiolucency between PA areas of max. centrals along the incisive canal	
Mandibular median cyst	Unilocular, in lower midline, separation of lower centrals	
Globulo-maxillary	Unilocular, pear shaped, between max lateral and canine root	
Mucus retention cyst in max sinus	Ovoid, at inferior extension of the floor of sinus	

RADIOLUCENT LESIONS OF JAWS

Lesions at apex of tooth	Soap bubble like R/L	Lesions in midline maxilla
Dental granuloma	Multilocular cyst	Median palatine cyst
Radicular cyst	Aneurysmal bone cyst	Median alveolar cyst
Residual cyst	Ameloblastoma	Globulomaxillary cyst
Periapical / DA abscess	Central GC granuloma	Nasoalveolar cyst
Apical scar	Cherubism, early stage	Incisive canal cyst
Cementoma (1st stage)	Myxoma/ non-odontogenic	Cyst of palatine papilla

Radiolucent Lesions of Jaws (*Contd.*)

Lesion in place of missing tooth	**Lesion around crown of impacted tooth**	**Multiple but separate R/L lesions**
Primordial cyst	Dentigerous cyst Ameloblastoma	Cherubism/early stage Multiple myeloma
Lesion that destroy cortical plate	Odontogenic adenomatoid tumor/ adenoameloblastoma	Eosinophilic granuloma
Metastatic tumor	Odontogenic fibroma and myxoma	Hand-Schuller – Christian disease
Primary malignant tumor		Letterer-Siwe disease
Osteomyelitis		Hyperpara- thyroidism/brown node/giant cell lesion Metastatic tumor

Miscellaneous R/L	**Partly R/O and partly R/L lesions of the jaw**	
Lateral PD cyst	Cementoma, 2nd stage	Condensing osteitis
Traumatic cyst	Ameloblastic fibro- odontoma	Chronic Sclerosing osteomyelitis
Idiopathic bone cavity	Cystic odontoma	
Osteomyelitis	Ossifying fibroma	
Hematopoietic marrow	Osteogenic sarcoma	

Radiolucent Lesions of Jaws (*Contd.*)

Gingival cyst	Chondrosarcoma	
Physiologic osteoporosis	Metastasis from ca. of prostate or breast	
Hemangioma/ central	Paget's disease	

RADIOPAQUE LESIONS OF THE JAWS

Cementoma	Chondrosarcoma
Root fragment/ foreign body	Condensing osteitis
Compound odontoma	Metastatic tumor
Complex odontoma	Paget's dis
Ossifying fibroma	Osteopetrosis
Fibrous dysplasia	Leontiasis ossea
Osteoma and torus	Caffey's disease
Osteogenic sarcoma	Garre's osteomyelitis
	Ch. sclerosing osteomyelitis

DISEASES OF THE BONE

Syndrome	Features
Osteogenesis imperfecta/brittle bone/ lobstein's disease	• Defect of *mesodermal tissues,* in organic matrix • Fragile bones, defective dentin, blue sclera • Basic defect: failure of collagen to mature
Infantile cortical hyperostosis/ Caffey's disease	• Due to local defect in blood supply • Arises during first 3 months of life • Mandible and clavicle affected most, deformity in ramal/angle region of mandible

Diseases of the Bone (*Contd.*)

Syndrome	Features
	• Increased serum alk Pase • R/G: sclerosis of cortex due to actively proliferating periosteum
Cleidocranial dysplasia/ Marie–Sainton disease	• Open fontanelles, sunken sagittal suture, • Underdeveloped maxilla (class III) • Prolonged retention of primary teeth • Multiple impacted, supernumerary teeth. • Absence / paucity of cellular cementum
Craniofacial dysostosis/ Crouzon's synd	• Crouzon's synd = no syndactyly • Apert's synd = with syndactyly • Early synostosis of sutures triangular frontal defect, exophthalmos, • Hypoplastic maxilla (class III), parrot-beak nose
Mandibulofacial dysostosis/ Treacher – Collins syndrome (eye, ear, face affected)	• Due to retardation/failure of differentiation of max. mesoderm at and after 50 mm embryo, after 2 mo. IU. • BILATERAL bird/fish like facies, PNS underdeveloped • Hypoplastic malar/mandible, class II m.o • Malformed ears/anti-mongoloid palpebral fissure • D/D = Goldenhar's syndrome (hemifacial microsomia, oculo-auriculo-vertebral dysplasia) is UNILATERAL, due to abnormal blood supply of head
Pierre Robin syndrome/ Robin anomalad	TRIAD = Cleft palate + micrognathia + glossoptosis Primary Defect = arrested development of mandible Bird-facies, cleft lip (CL) does not occur with cleft palate (CP).

Diseases of the Bone (*Contd.*)

Syndrome	Features
	Class II m.o, challenging dental treatment
Marfan synd/ arachnodactyly	Defective organisation of collagen, it is abnormally soluble, Excessive length of tubular bones, **Spidery fingers**, dolichofacial, hyperextensive joints, High palate, multiple odontogenic cysts, Class III m.o
Downs synd / trisomy 21 /	Most common chromosomal disorder, Translocation = 21 chr. material goes to chr. of G or D group, Increases with mother's age Class III m.o, mand. prognathism, macroglossia, Ass. with leukemia ALL, Complete freedom from caries
Osteopetrosis/ marble bone dis/ Albers – Schonberg dis	Diffuse sclerosis of many bones Most common C/F=optic atrophy (2,7,8 N compression) Pathological fractures / chances of osteomylitis after extractions (decreased medullary spaces). More caries, retarded eruption, R/G = diffuse sclerosis of bones so roots of teeth are nearly invisible. Lab = myelophthisic anemia, increased acid P ase,
Achondroplasia Paget's dis/ osteitis	Disturbed endochondral bone formation, = dwarfism Retarded maxillary growth = class III m.o, Disturbance of epiphyseal C of bones • Bones are excessively vascular, warm to touch, fragile

Diseases of the Bone (*Contd.*)

Syndrome	Features
deformans	• Slow virus / infection may be the cause • Progressive enlargement of skull, increased alk. Pase • Deafness (due to pressure on cochlear N) • Blindness (due to pressure on optic N) • Facial palsy (due to pressure on facial N) • Simian appearance, maxilla larger than mandible, progressive denture tightness, • R/G: **cotton wool appearance**, • Loss of normal trabeculations, bilateral disease, hypercementosis, loss of well defined lamina dura • H/E = mosaic bone, **jig saw puzzle appearance** • Treatment = calcitonin, (PTH antagonist), mithramycin
Vanishing bone/ Massive osteolysis/ phantom bone	Due to active hyperemia of bones, pathological fractures, H/E= <u>no osteoclasts</u> (it is a very striking feature from other areas of bone resorption)
Fibrous dysplasia	1. Jaffe's type = FD + café- au-lait spots 2. Albright synd = polyostotic FD + pigmentation + endocrine disturbances. 3. Pigmentation = is ka Café- au- lait spots; their margins are irregular resembling a map of COAST LINE OF MAIME. C/F = unilateral involvement, deformity of bones, café- au lait spots, precocious puberty only in females; teeth involved are not displaced and no root resorption is seen; HOCKEY-STICK DEFORMITY = leg length discrepancy due to involvement of upper part of femur;

Diseases of the Bone (*Contd.*)

Syndrome	Features
	R/G = multilocular cystic appearance, rarefied medullary portion, increased BMR, and Alk. Pase. R/G of skull = increased density of base of skull; i.e. occiput, sella turcica; roof of orbit and frontal bone. It is the most characteristic R/G feature of FD of skull. • Malignant transformation in **osteosarcoma** if treated by radiation therapy, i.e. post-radiation bone sarcoma. So radiation is C/I • **Leontiasis ossea** = because of lion like appearance, FD involving facial bones giving leonine's appearance. • R/G = ground glass/ peau-de-orange appearance, the margins are not well defined (cleft palate (cp) to ossifying fibroma which has well defined margins) • H/E = thin cortices but non-perforated, immature, irregular trabeculae arranged in curvilinear shapes as **Chinese character pattern or Chinese script writing** and C-shaped, • In most cases, the disease tends to stabilise and essentially stops growing when skeletal maturation is reached. Rx is by parring / shaving of bone for cosmetics.
Cherubism	**Bilateral**, familial, 3–4 yrs children which look like PLUMP CHEEKED LITTLE ANGELS, mostly in mandible, bone expansion and extensive destruction. • Premature shedding of deciduous teeth, delayed permanent tooth eruption; partial anodontia of permanent teeth,

Diseases of the Bone (*Contd.*)

Syndrome	Features
	• R/G = multilocular appearance, severe thin cortices with perforation, (cp from fibrous dysplasia) • **Teeth floating** in cyst like spaces, • H/E = multinuclear giant cells (MNGC), lesions are indistinguishable from central giant cell granuloma of jaws. Perivascular eosinophilic cuffing of capillaries; • Normal alk Pase; Ca; P serum levels • Becomes static/ regresses with onset of puberty • Radiation therapy is contraindicated.
Still's dis	Rheumatic arthritis in children involving TMJ and causing Class II div. I m.o
Ankylosis bilateral	Class II m.o

DISEASES OF SKIN

Hereditary ectodermal dysplasia	**Ectodermal tissue** affected, e.g. hypohidrosis, hypotrichosis, hypodontia, defective sebaceous and sweat glands Inability to endure warm temperature. Depressed nose, growth of jaws not impaired.
Chondro-ectodermal dysplasia	**Ectodermal tissues** affected, but **sweat mechanism is normal**, bilateral polydactyly, mid part of **upper lip fused** to upper gingival margin to eliminate normal mucogingival sulcus.
Lichen planus	Lesions bilateral, on **flexor** surfaces. **Wickham's striae,**

Diseases of Skin (*Contd.*)

	Ig and complements present at **epidermal-dermal junction** of skin Liquefaction degeneration of basal cells **Grinspan synd** = LP + D. mellitus + Hypertension H/E= acanthosis, intracellular oedema of spinous cells Saw-tooth like rete-pegs/ **civatte bodies** in epithelial cells • Lymphocytic infiltration sharply limited to PAPILLARY layer and most superficial part of reticular layer, i.e. SUBEPITHELIAL LYMPHOCYTIC AGGREGATION • Arifactual tearing between epith. and CT • Malignant potential = to SCC • Florescence which outlines basement membrane zone with numerous irregular extensions in superficial lamina propria = seen in lichen and lupus erythematosus. • Patchy linear pattern of fluorescence = in pemphigoid, erythema multiforme, • Granular pattern = in pemphigus,
Psoriasis	**Auspitz's sign** = lesions covered with silvery scales/ mica, Involve **extensor** surface, severe in winters. Polygenic inheritance, associated with HLA complex, increased serum IgG, A, cAMP, cGMP. H/E = absent **str granulosum**, elongation and clubbing of rete pegs. **Monro's abcess** (intraepithelial), perivascular and periadnexal lymphocytic and histiocytic infiltration. Very rapid rate of skin epithelial turnover, increased mitosis.

Diseases of Skin (*Contd.*)

Pityriasis rosea	Primary lesion is called as **herald spot**, ovoid shaped with long axis parallel to natural lines of cleavage of skin, seldom recurs.
Erythema multiforme/ Stevens – Johnson synd Darrier's dis / keratosis follicularis	**Target/ iris/ bull's eye** lesions. It involves skin/ oral cavity/eyes/ genitalia. H/E = intracellular oedema of spinous layer & oedema of superficial CT, SUBEPIDERMAL VESICLES, intraepithelial vesicles formation. Toxic epidermal necrolysis **(Lyell's dis)**= drug eruptions Related to vit. A metabolism H/E = CORPS ROND and GRAINS, found just above the basal layer of cells, i.e. SUPRABASILAR CLEAVAGE. Peculiar hyperplasia of epith. rests of Malassez in PDL. Basic defect = in desmosome-tonofilament complex seven times decrease in turnover time of epithelium, as **psoriasis**
Incontinenta pigmenti	**Hallmark of synd** = Heavy melanin pigmentation of epith dropping down in clusters of chromatophores in upper dermis Lethal to males, marked eosinophilia. Delayed eruption, missing and malformed teeth
Dyskeratosis congenita	**Males only,** *triad* = leucoplakia, dystrophy of nails, skin pigmentation High incidence of oral cancer/malignant transformation **Fanconi's anemia**/ synd may be associated.
White sponge nevus/ Cannon's dis	Cells of spinous layer show intracellular edema. Familial,

Diseases of Skin (*Contd.*)

Acanthosis nigrans	**Hypertrophy of filiform papillae** of tongue
Pemphigus	Autoimmune disease, intercellular antibodies present. **Nikolsky's sign** = due to perivesicular edema disrupting dermal-epidermal junction. **Senear-usher synd** = lesions associated with crusted patches resembling seborrhic dermatitis. O/E = serpiginous pattern in mouth resembling pus. H/E = intraepithelial lesion, suprabasilar split, acantholysis, TZANCK CELLS. • **scarcity of inflammatory cell infiltration**, (cp to other bullous dis which have marked inflammation) • immunoflouresence test = IgG in intercellular spaces/ substance
Hailey- Hailey dis/familial benign chronic pemphigus	Epidermal defect, in desmosome- tonofilament complex, NIKOLSKY'S sign positive, more extensive acantholysis (cp to pemphigus), but not entirely acantholytic = DILAPIDATED BRICK WALL APPEARANCE
Cicatrical pemphigoid	Lesions esp **near body orifices**. Eye = obliteration of palpebral fissure due to adhesion of palpebral and bulbar conjuctiva. H/E = lesions are SUBEPIDERMAL, no acantholysis. Immunoflouresence = tissue bound basement membrane zone antibodies
Bullous pemphigoid/ parapemphigus	Subepidermal lesions, no acantholysis. Altered penetrability of blood vessels. Circulating basement membrane antibodies
Epidermolysis bullosa	Lesions due to destruction of basal/ suprabasal cells

Diseases of Skin (*Contd.*)

	EB dystrophic, recessive = bullae immediately below basement memb, + ve nikolsky sign, pre-elastic and oxytalan fibres increased in number. **Junctional EB** = 3 criteria = onset at birth, absence of scarring, death within 3 mos age.
Dermatitis herpetiformis	Associated with malabsorption enteropathy, villous atrophy of intestine. H/E= neutrophils and eosinophils in dermal papilla, microabscess. **Eosinophils** are very prominent and characteristic. Immunoflouresence = at epidermal- dermal junction, (only IgA) Patient is sensitive to halogens. Treatment = SULPHAPYRIDINE
Acrodermatitis enteropathica	Related to **Zn- malabsorption synd**, low serum Zn levels, deficient CMI
Lupus erythematosus/ SLE/ DLE	Autoimmune dis, butterfly lesions, F: M = 8:1. Kidneys= fibrinoid degeneration of glomeruli, **wire-loop pattern**. DLE= carpet-teck extensions in pilosebaceous canals, peripheral growth of lesions, scarring. SCC/BCC may develop. • **LE cells inclusion phenomenon** = rosette of neutrophils surrounding a pale nuclear mass derived from neutrophils, • +ve **Coomb's test**, increased ESR, • H/E= atrophy of rete- pegs, hyperkeratosis, absent keratinisation in SLE • Immunoflouresence = at dermal-epidermal junction, as particulate/speckled pattern

Diseases of Skin (*Contd.*)

Systemic sclerosis/ Hidebound's dis	Autoimmune/ thyroid/ parathyroid, as causes. Progressive fibrosis of skin, due to vascular insufficiency. RAYNAUD'S phenomenon = + ve. **Acrosclerosis**= SS+ Raynaud's dis + sclerosis of distal parts of extremities esp digits (sclerodactyly). C/F = fixation of epidermis to deeper CT, ivory-white waxy appearance, calcium deposition, fixed skin = mask like face, claw-like hands. **CREST synd** = calcinosis cutis + Raynaud's dis + oesophageal dysfunction + sclerodactyly + telengiectasia. MORPHEA = i.e. circumscribed scleroderma. **Coup-de-sabre** = linear scleroderma. O/E = stiff, board like tongue, decreased mouth opening. R/G = extreme widening of PDL due to increase in collagen and oxytalan fibres and hyalinisation of collagen, bone loss at mandibular angle. H/E= loss of dermal appendages esp sweat glands, epithelial atrophy, loss of rete pegs, increased melanin pigmentation.
Ehler's- Danlos synd/cutis hyper elastica	Abnormal collagen, hyperextensibility of joints, fragile skin, defective healing of wounds. In EDS –IV= rupture of large arteries and intestine may occur **Circus- rubberman patient.** Scars tend to spread rather than contract with time. Fragile MM = does not hold sutures Lack of normal scalloping of DEJ, increased pulp stones
Focal dermal hypoplasia	Mesoectodermal dysplasia. Focal absence of dermis, herniation of s/c fat.

Diseases of Skin (*Contd.*)

synd/ Goltz-Gorlin synd	Pappillomas of lips and skin, microdontia
Solar elastosis	Degenerative skin called as SAILOR'S SKIN,/ farmer's skin. Increased elastic CT fibres. Basophilic degeneration of CT

TYPICAL RADIOGRAPHIC FEATURES

Ball-in-hand appearance	Benign salivary gland tumors
Balloon- like appearance	Follicular cyst, aneurysmal bone cyst
Candle-stick appearance	Pyknodysostosis, progressive systemic sclerosis
Chalk-like appearance	Osteopetrosis, hyperparathyroidism, pykno-dysostosis
Cherry-blossom pattern	Sjogren's synd, mikulicz dis
Codman's triangle	Osteosarcoma
Cotton-wool appearance	Fibrous dysplasia, odontogenic fibroma, paget's dis
Egg-shell appearance	Ameloblastoma, multilocular cyst
Filling defect	Salivary gland tumor
Floating tooth appearance	SCC of gingiva, malignant lymphoma, cherubism, eosinophilic granuloma, burkit's lymphoma
Ground glass appearance	Fibrous dysplasia, ossifying fibroma, osteosarcoma, hyperparathyroidism

Typical Radiographic Features (*Contd.*)

Hair-on-end appearance	Central hemangioma, Paget's dis
HONEYCOMB appearance	Ameloblastoma, central hemangioma
Moth-eaten appearance	SCC of gingiva, malignant lymphoma, chronic osteomylitis, histiocytosis-X, tumor-degeneration of condyle, eosinophilic granuloma
Mottled appearance	Fibrous dysplasia, ossifying fibroma
Onion-peel appearance	Chronic osteomylitis, eosinophilic granuloma, Ewing's sarcoma
Permeated type	Carcinoma of gingiva, SCC of maxilla, malignant lymphoma
Pear-shaped appearance	Globulomaxillary cyst, radicular cyst
Pencil-line appearance	Ameloblastoma, traumatic bone cyst, CEOC, i.e. gorlin cyst
Pressure-type appearance	SCC of gingiva
Punched-out appearance	Multiple myeloma; Hand–Schuller–Christian disease
Sand-like appearance	Adenoameloblastoma, CEOC, CEOT, i.e. pindborg tumor
Salt and pepper appearance	Hyperparathyroidism, traumatic bone cyst, aneurysmal bone cyst, giant-cell granuloma
Scalloping pattern	Dentigerous cyst, traumatic bone cyst, aneurysmal bone cyst, giant-cell tumor
Soap-bubble appearance	Ameloblastoma, giant-cell granuloma, central hemangioma
Spiked root	Malignant histiocytoma, Burkitt lymphoma

Typical Radiographic Features (*Contd.*)

Sun-ray appearance	Osteosarcoma,
Tennis-racket appearance	Odontogenic myxoma
Worm-eaten/moth-eaten appearance	Carcinoma of gingiva, malignant lymphoma, chronic osteomylitis
Hanging drop sign	
Salt and pepper effect in MRI	Sjogren's synd
Step ladder effect in PA view	Sickle cell anemia
Tram line appearance on face	In CSF rhinnorhea
Bifid mandibular canal	Neurofibromatosis

MOST COMMONS

Benign oral cancer	Fibroma
Cleft lip	Unilateral complete
Fissural cyst	Median anterior palatine cyst
Malignant tumor of major salivary glands	Adenocarcinoma
Malignant tumor of salivary glands in post palatal area	Adenoid cystic car. It spreads along perineurial sheath.
Metastatic lesion to jaw bones is from a primary tumor located in	Breast
Nevus	Intradermal
Odontogenic cyst	Radicular cyst
Odontogenic tumor	Ameloblastic fibroma

Most Commons (*Contd.*)

Site of SCC	Lower lip near mucocutaneous junction
Supernumerary tooth	Mesiodens
Tumor of oral mucosa	SCC
Tumor of parotid	Pleomorphic adenoma
Viral infection	Herpes simplex

TYPICAL FEATURES

Dick test	For scarlet fever D for S
Frei's test	for lymphogranuloma venerum
FTA test (not VDRL)	Specific for syphilis
Kveim –Siltzbach's test	Sarcoidosis
Positive Paul- Bunnel test	Infectious mononucleosis
Schilling test	For vit B_{12} absorption
Shick test	Diphtheria S for D
Weil-Felix test	Rickettesial infection, lymphogranuloma venerum
Anitschkow cells	Recurrent aphthae / canker sores
Antoni type A, B bodies, Varocay body	Neurilemmoma,
Argyll Robertson pupil	Neurosyphilis
Aschoff's body	Rheumatic fever, heart dis
Auspitz sign	Psoriasis
Bitot's spots	Vit A deficiency

Typical Features (*Contd.*)

Carpet-tack extensions	Erythema multiforme
Cori's abscess	TB
Corps and ronds	Keratosis follicularis
Crushman's spirals	In sputum of asthmatic patient
Cytoid body and Civette body	L. planus
Donovan body	Granuloma inguinale
Fordyce's granules	Ectopic sebaceous glands
Fordyce's spots	Ectopic sebaceous glands
Guarnieri body	Small pox
Haberden's nodes	Osteoarthritis
Handerson- Paterson / molluscum body	Molluscum contagiosum
Heart failure cells of lungs	Phagocytic cells having hemosiderin
Hebra nose	Rhinoscleroma
Herald's spots	Cardinal sign of pityriasis rosea
Iris/bull eye/ target lesions	Erythema multiforme
Koplik's spots	In measles/ rubeola
Langhans giant cells	TB
Lipschultz bodies/ Cowdery –A body	Herpes infection, primary. Herpetic stomatitis
Mallory body	Cirrhosis of liver; in liver cells

Typical Features (*Contd.*)

Monro's abscess	Psoriasis (it is least likely to show oral symptoms)
Negri's body	Rabies
Nikolsky's sign	Bullous pemphigoid
Pseudorhagades	Ectodermal dysplasia
Reed- Sternberg cells	Hodgkin's dis
Rushton body	Radicular cyst, any inflammatory cyst
Russel body	Multiple myeloma, chronic inflammation
Saddle nose	syphilis
Safety pin cells	Thalessemia in blood
Saw tooth rete pegs	L. planus
Tzank cells	Pemphigus, H. zoster
Warthen-Frenkeldey giant cells	Measles
Wickham striae	Lichen planus
Zanker's degeneration	Hyaline degeneration of voluntary Ms

Tuberculosis: pulmonary TB is the chief form of disease.

1. Phithisis = TB of lungs
2. Scrofula = TB of lymph nodes
3. Lupus vulgaris = TB of skin
4. Cori's abscess = in TB
5. Pott's dis =TB of spine, aka cervical caries
6. Miliary TB = if spreads by blood
7. Cold abscess = formed by TB

INCLUSION BODIES

1. Cytoplasmic = in pox virus, rabies, molluscum cantangiosum
2. Nuclear = in herpes virus, polio virus
3. Both = in measles, CMV disease

CONDITIONS OF TONGUE

Atrophic or interstitial glossitis	Syphilis
Bald tongue of Sandwith	Pellagra
Beefy red tongue	Niacin deficiency
Glosopyrosis	Burning tongue
Glossodynia	Painful tongue
Glossoplegia	Paralysis of tongue
Hairy tongue	Filiform papillae enlarge
Hunter's/Moeller's glossitis	Pernicious anemia
Magenta color tongue	Riboflavin, B_2 deficiency
Strawberry tongue	Scarlet fever (due to fungiform papillae)

CT diseases, e.g. SLE, rheumatoid arthritis, show hypergammaglobulinemia, i.e. increased antibodies.

Rheumatoid factor = an IgM antibody against host IgG.

Congenital syphilis affects the fetus = after 5 mos. IU

Acute angioedema = may be caused by C1- esterase deficiency, managed by DANZOL (a hormone, androgen)

HEPATITIS

- Hep-B is caused by viral particle ka Dane particle,
- HBs Ag = is Australia Ag, is DIAGNOSTIC; HbcAg = DNA containing core

- Anti HBs Ag and anti HBc Ag presence show that patient is immune to Hep-B and can be treated as no- Hep risk.
- HbeAg is more infective than HBs Ag.
- Hep-B immune globulin = gives passive and transient immunity
- Hep- B infection in adult is = subclinical
- 5.2 % NaOCl is effective vs Hep-B virus for sterilisation.

LEVELS

- Increased serum alk Pase = paget's disease, pregnancy, adolescence., von-Recklinghausen's disease of bone (primary Hyperparathyroidism, increased serum Ca^{++}), infantile cortical hyperostosis ·
- Decreased serum alk Pase = hypophosphatasia
- Increased serum acid Pase = jaw metastatis of prostatic cancer
- Increased serum IgG, IgA = psoriasis
- Multiple myeloma = inceased Ca, decreased PO_4, normal alk. Pase in serum
- Paget's dis = Increased serum alk Pase, normal Ca, PO_4, urinary hydroxyproline excretion

	Ca	P	Alk. Pase
Hyperparathyroidism	Increased	Decreased	Increased
Paget's dis	N	N	Increased
Multiple myeloma	Increased	Decreased	N

Staining of teeth

1. Blue green brown = erythroblastosis fetalis; due to bilirubin
2. Purplish red = porphyria
3. Yellow = cystic fibrosis
4. Yellow brown = tetracycline (occurs in dentin, can not be treated by bleaching)

5. White-brown = flouride, occurs in enamel, bleaching gives good results.
6. Plumbism = basophilic stippling of RBCs.

VITAMINS: fat soluble = A, D, E, K; water soluble = B, C

Vitamin	Synonym	Adult daily req	Deficiency
A	Retinol	750 μg	• Xerophthalmia/night blindness • Helps ameloblast integrity maintenance
C	Ascorbic acid	40 mg	Deficiency primarily affects the tissues of mesenchymal origin; Scurvy
E	Tocopherol, antioxidant	10 IU	
D	Calciferol	100 units	Rickets/ osteomalacia
K	Naphthoquinone	—	
B_1	Thiamine	1.2 mg	Beri-beri
B_2	Riboflavin	1.7 mg	Angular chielosis
B_3	Pantothenic acid	10 mg	
B_6	Pyridoxine	1.5 mg	Hypochromic, microcytic anemia
B_{12}	Cyanocobalamine	1 μg	Macrocytic/pernicious anemia
H	Biotin	—	
	Niacin	18 mg	Pellagra
	Intrinsic factor		Pernicious anemia
	Folic acid	100 μg	Megaloblastic anemia
	Chronic blood loss		Microcytic, hypochromic anemia

INFECTIONS

Condition	Cause	Clinical Features
Scarlet fever	Beta-hemolytic streptococci, erythrogenic toxins	Skin rashes due to injury to vascular endothelium and hyperemia; hyperemic papillae so *strawberry tongue*; coating of tongue lost, so *raspberry tongue*
Diphtheria	*Corynebacterium diphtheriae*; aka Klebs-Loefller bacillus	Diphtheric membrane, soft palate temporarily paralysed; nasal twang
TB	*Mycobacterium tuberculosis*, AFB	Ulcers have undermined edges; tongue esp base most commonly affected; U/L jaws involved by anachoretic effect in areas of PA inflammation forming tuberculoma. H/E = caseous necrosis
Sarcoidosis	Granulomatous dis	Depressed delayed hypersensitivity i.e. **CMI**; increased abnormal serum IgG; lymphoproliferation; H/E= resembles TB, but no caseous necrosis; no AFB
Uveoparotid fever/ Heerfordt's synd	A form of sarcoidosis	Bilateral parotid swelling; Inflammed uveal tract of eyes; 7th N involvement
Leprosy/ Hansen's dis	*Mycobacterium laprae*/ AFB	Involve dermal and peripheral N trunks; loss of sensations; H/E= **lepra cells** = vacuolated *macrophages;* contain bacilli
Actinomycosis/ray fungus	Actinomyces israelii; G +, non AFB,	**Sulphur granules** = colonies of bacteria,Cervicofacial actinomycosis= commonest

Infections (*Contd.*)

	anaerobes	**Ray fungus appearance** of bacterial filament
Botryomycosis actinobacillosis	Granulomatous	
Tularemia/ rabbit fever	*Pasteurella tularenesis*	Eyes, lymph nodes involved
Melioidosis	*Pseudomonas mallei*	Lung, LNs, sinus, visceral involvement
Tetanus/ lock jaw	*Clostridium tetani*, exotoxins, anaerobes, G +	Intense activity of motor neurons; severe muscle spasm; Exotoxins act on synapses of interneurons of inhibitory pathways and motor neurons = block spinal inhibition, C/F= lock jaw/trismus; stiffness of jaw/neck ms., **risus sardonicus,** i.e. rigid facial ms., **opisthotonus,** i.e. entire body ms affected; **cephalic tetanus,** i.e. mostly 7 th N palsy
Syphilis/lues	*Treponema pallidum*/seen best by darkfield microscopy in silver impregnation, affects oral structures if encountered in second trimester of pregnancy	(A) Acquired =3 stages; primary/secondary are infectious/painless; • **primary = chancre**; after 3 weeks at inoculation site; heals spontaneously in 3 wk-2 mo. time; intense inflammatory infilterate esp plasma cells; • **secondary** = is metastatic stage; after 6 wk of primary

Infections (*Contd.*)

		lesions, ka **mucous patches,** on tongue, gingiva, etc. or as a split papule on lips, highly infectious; serologic reaction is always positive; Infections • tertiary = **late syphilis; gumma;** is a granuloma with central necrosis; non-infectious; after many years; most common on tongue, palate; palatal perforation by ulcer after vigorous antibiotic use, ka **Herxheimer reaction** • atrophic/ **interstitial glossitis** is most characteristic lesion = has malignant potential to SCC. **(B) congenital/ prenatal** = most constant finding is relatively short roots of mandibular. Permanent. First molars; treatment should be started before 4 mo. IU. C/F = short maxilla; **class III**; saddle nose; **Higoumenakis's sign** i.e. irregular thickening of sternoclavicular part on clavicle. Dish face deformity. **Hutchinson's triad** = teeth/ eye/ ear involved. • hypoplasia of incisors and molars i.e. notched (screwdriver shaped) incisors and mulberry/ moon's/ Fournier's molars

Infections (*Contd.*)

		• eighth nerve deafness • interstitial keratitis
Granuloma inguinale/ donovanosis	*Calymmato-bacterium* granulomatis	**Donovan bodies** in tissue of lesion. Ulcers with rolled margins showing peripheral enlargement tendency. Inguinal ulceration as fluctuant swelling ka pseudobubo. H/E = pathognomic; p.o. large mononuclear phagocytes, each having tiny intracytoplasmic cysts, containing donovan bodies. Cicatrization = most C/F of oral lesions
Lympho-granuloma venerum	*Chlamydia trachomatis*	No oral lesions
Rhino-scleroma	*Klebsiella rhinoscleromatis* type 3	Hebra nose
Midline lethal granuloma		Localised progressive destruction of nose, PNS, palate, face, etc. Is due to dysfunction of immune mech. (periarteritis nodosa, Arthus reaction), Obstructed blood supply and necrosis
Wegner's granulo-matosis	Hypersensitivity reaction to unknown antigen	Is a systemic dis, involves vascular, renal, resp. system. H/E = giant cell granulomatous lesions

Infections (*Contd.*)

Chronic granulo-matous dis	Defects of intracellular leucocyte enzyme functions, decreased oxidative metabolism, failure to destroy catalase + ve microorganism	H/E = mononuclear histiocytes, MNGC Diagnosis = failure to reduce nitroblue tetrazolium i.e. NBT test
Noma / cancrum oris	Gangrenous stomatitis, by vincent's organism	ANUG
Pyogenic granuloma	*Staph./ Strept.*	SH radical is most essential stimulating agent.
Regional enteritis/ ileitis	Aka Crohn's dis.	Granulomatous inflammation of of intestine
Pyostomatitis vegetans	Due to GIT disturbences	**Cobblestone appearance** of buccal mucosa; treated by salazopyrine

VIRAL INFECTIONS

Condition	Cause	Features
Herpes simplex / cold sores	HSV 1, VZV, EBV, CMV Primary infection = in patients having Abs produced	Most common; affects ecto-dermal tissues; produce Abs in blood; viral DNA gets incor-porated in host DNA; life long infection beyond the reach of Abs, CMI; drugs;

Viral Infections (*Contd.*)

Condition	Cause	Features
	by the virus in blood	Subclinical primary infection is common; HSV 2 is associated with ca. Uterine cervix; HSV does not remain latent at site of original infection; reaches regional ganglia along the nerve path; HSV 1 in trigeminal and HSV 2 in lumbosacral; H/E = intra-epithelial vesicles; balloning degeneration; intranuclear inclusions ka lipschultz bodies, i.e. **cowdry A type**, perinuclear halo in nucleus
Recurrent / sec. Herpes labialis	More in patients without Abs to HSV 1,2	Lesions on mucosa tightly-bound to periosteum; (aphthous on loose mucosa) H/E = papanicoulaou smear for diagnosis; Tzanck cells, **lipschultz bodies,** balloning degeneration; Rx = idoxuridine inhibits replication of HSV by irreversibly inhibiting the incorporation of thymidine in viral DNA; Arginine-rich diets cause recurrence of HSV infection Lysine = antagonist to arginine, so oral intake of lysine resolves HSV infection
Herpetic whitow		Recurrent lesions on fingers/ hands

Viral Infections (*Contd.*)

Condition	Cause	Features
Recurrent aphthous stomatitis/ canker sores	Strep. sanguis, L- form of alpha-hemolytic strept.	Delayed hypersensitivity to S.sanguis and altered immune response; Auto-immune response of oral epith. = IgG, M binding by spinous epith cells of oral mucosa. Ulcers occur on mobile mucosa; H/E = **anitschkow cells**
Sutton's dis		Periadenitis mucosa necrotica recurrence aka **mikulicz's scarring**
Behcet's synd	PPLO virus; autoimmune	HLA differentiates b/w it & rec.aphthous ulcers, increased auto-Abs to mucosa C/F= triad = rec.oral and genital ulcers; ocular inflammation; skin lesions
Reiter's synd	PPLO, bedsonia group virus	**Tetrad** = arthritis, mucocutaneous lesions, urithritis and conjunctivitis (AMUC) Arthritis is bilateraaly symmetrical and polyarticular
Herpangina	Coxsackie A virus	Ulcers on anterior faucial pillars, palate, post. pharynx; a permanent immunity develops to the infecting strains rapidly–Abs found. Animal inoculation of virus causes destruction of skeletal ms. and death

Viral Infections (*Contd.*)

Condition	Cause	Features
Acute Lympho-nodular pharyngitis	Coxsackie virus A 10	Lesions consist of densly packed nodules of lymphocytes
HFM dis	Enterovirus coxsackie A 16	In young children, intracy-toplasmic viral inclusions
FM dis/ aphthous fever	Only in animals, rarely in man	Transmitted by infected milk
Measles/ rubeola	Paramyxo virus	Portal of entry = respiratory tract C/F = skin eruptions-blanch on ressure O/F = **Koplik's spots** = pro-dromal and pathognomic; immu-nosuppressive
Rubella/ german measles	Myxovirus, affects oral structures if encountered in first trimester of pregnancy	**No Koplik's spots**; if occurs during first trimester of pre-gnancy = causes congenital defects
Smallpox/ variola	Pox virus	
Molluscum contagiosum	Pox group virus	Nodules in eyelid; umblicated in centre; H/E = intracytolasmic inclusion bodies aka **Handerson –Pater-son inclusions** aka molluscum bodies;

Viral Infections (*Contd.*)

Condition	Cause	Features
Condyloma acuminatum	Veneral wart by HPV/ HPV 6	
Chicken pox/ varicella	VZV	Inflammation of dorsal nerve root ganglia or extramedullary cranial n. ganglia, i.e. sensory nerves,— is always unilateral, Intranuclear inclusion bodies and MNGC (tzanck cells) • primary. Infection with VZV = chicken pox • sec. infection = herpes zoster
Hunt's synd/ Ramsay Hunt's synd	VZV	Infection of geniculate ganglion, involved external ear & oral M.Memb.; facial paralysis
Cat-scratch dis		Oculoglandular synd of Parinaud = localised granulomas of eye and periauricular LAP
Mumps/ parotitis	Paramyxovirus	Mostly bilateral swelling of parotids; Orchitis is main complication. Increased serum lipase, amylase due to pancreas involvement;
Cytomegalic inclusion dis	CMV, it also causes CMV mononucleosis & Kaposi's sarcoma in AIDS	Most common viral cause of mental retardation. Intranuclear and cytoplasmic inclusions in cells of salivary glands = pathognomic
Polio		Ganglia involved

Anitschkow cells: also found in:

- sickle cell disease
- canker sores
- megaloblastic anemia
- iron-deficiency anemia
- pts on chemotherapy

FUNGAL INFECTIONS

Condition	Cause	Features
Gilchrist's dis/American blastomycosis	*Blastomyces dermatitidis*	Resembles SCC, is granulomatous infection; giant cells contain microorganisms; mostly in dogs, outdoor workers
Lutz's dis/ south American blasto-/ paracoccidioidomycosis	*B. brasilienesis/ paracoccidioides*	
Darling's disease/ histoplasmosis	*Histoplasma capsulatum*	By **inhalation of excreta of birds,** e.g. pigeon; involves RE system; pulmonary calcified nodules, so confused with TB; org. is found intracellularly in phagocytes
Coccidioidomycosis/ valley fever	*Coccidioides immitis*	By inhalation of *dust* having spores; chronic granulomatous lesion; coagulation necrosis; MNGC having the microorg.
Cryptococcosis/ European blastomycosis	*Cryptococcus neoformans / C. bacillispora*	Lesions involve meninges; harboured by pigeons; org. appears as tissue- microcysts; MNGCs are present;

Fungal Infections (*Contd.*)

Condition	Cause	Features
Candidiasis/ moniliasis/ thrush	*Candida albicans*	Most oppurtunistic infection in the world; impaired CMI, IgA deficiency; **White plaques** = can be wiped away (leucoplakia plaques can not be) Chronic form = aka denture sore mouth Hyphae / yeast cells are seen in superficial layers of involved epithelium
Phycomy-cosis/ mucormy-cosis	*Phycomycetes* orgs. i.e. rhizopus, mucor, absidia	Oppurtunistic infection esp in **diabetes mellitus** (diabetic ketoacidosis) Syndrome = uncontrolled diabetes, cellulitis, ophthalmoplegia, meningoencephlitis Thrombus formation and necrosis
Sporo-trichosis	*Sporotrichum schenckii*	Sporotrichotic chancres, granulomatous reactions, asteroid bodies

DEVELOPMENTAL SYNDROMES

Aamilial	Absence of fungiform and circumvallate papillae and taste buds; taste deficit
Ascher's synd	Acquired double lips + blepharochalosis + nontoxic thyroid enlargement
Atresia	Congenital absence / occlusion of one/ more of major salivary glands ducts; v. rare

Developmental Syndromes (*Contd.*)

Beckwith's hypoglycemic synd	Macroglossia; neonatal hypoglycemia; mild microcephaly; umbilical hernia; fetal visceromegaly; postnatal somatic giantism
Benign migratory glossitis/ geographic tongue	Multiple areas without filiform papillae; but fungiform papillae persist;
Branchial cyst	Lymphoepithelial cyst, from cystic transformation of glandular epithelium during embryogenesis; at floor of mouth or ventral tongue
Cheilitis glandularis	Enlarged labial salivary glands and inflammed orifices; males; lower lip
Congenital macroglossia	Due to overdevelopment of muscles
Ephelis	Melanotic macules; increased melanin in basal layers
Fissured/ scrotal tongue	Most common dev disorder of tongue; due to vit def.
Fordyce's granules	Sebaceous glands colections; on buccal mucosa opposite the upper molars; as yellow spots
Hairy tongue	Hypertrophy of filiform papillae; may be due to candida albicans
Heck's dis	Focal epithelial hyperplasia; mostly on lower lips; papova virus is the cause. H/E = acanthosis/ thickening of spinous layer; increased rete-pegs
Kimura's dis	Angiolymphoid eosinophilic hyperplasia
Lingual thyroid nodules	Thyroid anlage ramnants in tongue; thyroid gland dev. from ventral floor of pharynx by endodermal invagination or diverticulum

Developmental Syndromes (*Contd.*)

Macroglossia	In hyperpituitarism; cretinism, i.e. congenital hypothyroidism; tumors; lymphatic blockage; amyloidosis.
Macrognathia	In paget's dis (maxilla); leontiasis ossea (i.e. fibrous dysplasia; maxilla); gigantism/ acromegaly (mandible)
Median rhomboid glossitis	Congenital; failure of tuberculum impar to retract; area is devoid of filiform papilla; lie anterior to circumvallete papillae; common in diabetics due to candida albicans as cause; H/E = proliferation of spinous layer; elongation of rete pegs
Melkersson-Rosenthal synd	Triad = cheilitis granulomatosis + facial palsy + **scrotal tongue,** Chronic inflammatory cells infiltration = plasma cells, lymphocytes, histiocytes
Miescher's synd	Aka cheilitis granulomatosis,; swelling of lower lip
Parry- Romberg syndrome	Facial hemiatrophy, esp LHS of face is involved
Peutz-Jeghar's syndrome	Intestinal polyposis + pigmented face/ oral cavity/ limbs; Mostly Small intestine polyps; (cleft palate (cp) to Gardener's synd = large intestine polyps); polyps of colon = malignant tendency
Pierre-Robin Syndrome	Micrognathia
Reactive lymphoid aggregate	Lingual tonsils; located on post 1/3 rd of tongue; Aka foliate papilitis
Sjogren's synd	Xerostomia is due to destruction and atrophy of acinar tissues of salivary glands

Developmental Syndromes (*Contd.*)

Stafne cyst/ lingual mand salivary gland depression/ static bone cavity	Lies below mand canal; in mand 2 nd, 3 rd molar region anterior to angle. Traumatic bone cyst lies above the mand canal
Vander- Woude's	Pits of lower lip + CL/CP, lip pits develop from failure of complete union of embryonic lateral sulci of lips
Xerostomia	Etio.= Pernicious / iron- deficiency anemia; atropine; antihistaminic drugs; x rays; etc. Def. Of vit A = affects epithelium; produces squamous metaplasia; sicca syndrome (kerato-conjunctivitis sicca) Oral mucous membrane is pale/ dry/ atrophic/ thin; Tongue = atrophy of papillae; fissuring; cracking, rampant dental caries

DEVELOPMENTAL DISTURBANCES OF TEETH

Microdontia	• generalised = in pituitary dwarfism, rare • individual = most common is maxillary 2 and 8, peg lateral
Macrodontia	Pituitary gigantism, rare Localised = in hemihypertrophy of face.
Gemination	Due to incomplete division of tooth germ,; single root and RC.
Twinning	Div. of tooth germ to produce one normal and one supernumerary tooth.
Fusion	Union of two tooth germs; Completed if fusion occurs before calci-fication

Developmental Disturbances of Teeth (*Contd.*)

	Roots only if fusion occurs after crown completion; Dentin is always confluent; RC can be fused or separate.
Concrescence	Fusion after root completion i.e. of cementum
Dilaceration	Curve/ sharp bend in root; due to trauma
Talon's cusp	At lingual surface of permanent incisors; has a pulp horn; Common in **Rubinstein-Tayabi syndrome** = developmental retardation, broad toes, decrease bone age.
Dens-in dente/ dens invaginatus	Tooth in a tooth; Due to invagination in surface of crown before calcification; Mostly in maxillary lateral incisors; bilateral; accentuated lingual pit; Radicular invagination is due to infolding of Hertwig's root sheath Closely near the pulp and seen as pear-shaped in R/G;
Dens evaginatus	Accessory globule on occlusal surface of premolars; Due to proliferation and evagination of an area of *IEE* and mesenchyme into dental organ during early tooth development.
Taurodontism	Bull-like teeth; body of tooth enlarged at the expense of roots; By failure of Hertwig's root sheath to invaginate at proper horizontal level; very common in Neanderthal man; Found in Klinefelter's synd (males XXY) Mainly permanent molars are involved; Pulp chambers are very large and rectangular, RCs are v.v short

Developmental Disturbances of Teeth (*Contd.*)

Supernumarary roots	Mainly in mand. 3,4,5, 8 and maxillary 8
Anodontia	**Butler's field theory,** i.e. distal tooth of the groups is affected, e.g. 2,5,8; but in mand incisors, an exception exist where centrals are missing rather than laterals. • True = in hereditary ectodermal dysplasia; both deciduous/ permanent teeth affected. • Pseudo = multiple unerupted teeth. • Induced/ false = due to extractions • Partial = 8 > mand 5 > maxillary 5 > maxillary 2; congenitally missing deciduous teeth are rare (max B > mand B,C); is due to point mutations/ familial • Total = rare
Supernumerary teeth	Develop from 3 rd tooth bud/splitting of permanent tooth bud; Most common = mesiodens (maxillary), M> F,; autosomal dominant; 90% occur in maxilla; very less in deciduous teeth, (max B > max, mand C); Multiple supernumerary impacted teeth = in cleidocranial dysplasia
Gardener's synd	AD; single pleiotropic gene; 5 C/F = • multiple impacted supernumerary and permanent teeth • multiple polyposis of large intestine = premalignant • osteomas of bones • multiple epidermal/ sebaceous cysts • desmoid tumors
Pre-deciduous dentition	Are keratin-filled hornified epith structures without roots; should be removed, occur in **mand. incisors** area

Developmental Disturbances of Teeth (*Contd.*)

	Arise from an accessory bud of dental lamina ahead of deciduous bud or from bud of an accessory dental lamina; May be dental lamina cyst of newborn.
Natal teeth	True primary teeth at birth; should not be removed
Neonatal teeth	Erupt within 30 days of birth

A. AMELOGENESIS IMPERFECTA: ectodermal tissues affected,

1. **hypoplastic type** = in formative stage; defective organic matrix formation; enamel not fully formed;
2. **hypocalcified/ hypomineralised type** = in calcification stage; defective mineralisation of matrix; enamel is very soft; easily lost;
3. **hypomaturation type** = in maturation stage; immature crystals; enamel can be pierced by explorer under firm pressure and can be chipped away;
4. R/G: enamel is very thin/totally absent; open contacts/worn cusps.

B. ENAMEL HYPOPLASIA = occurs only during the formative stages;

1. Hereditary : both primary/permanent. Teeth involved; only enamel is affected;
2. Environmental = either primary or permanent teeth are involved; both E and D are affected; occurs due to injury and disturbance of ameloblasts;

Etiology =

1. **Vit A, C, D deficiency** = rickets, exanthematous disease, affect ameloblasts and metabolism, pitting type of EH occurs; teeth mostly formed during first year of life are afected i.e. 1,2,3 tip (tip starts dev. before dev. of 2) and 6. 4578 are not affected as they dev. after 3 years of age.
2. **Congenital syphilis** = EH not of pitting type, 126 are involved; aka <u>Hutchinson's incisors</u>; are notched; moon's/ mulberry/ Fournier

molars; incisors are screwdriver shape; tapered and notched due to absence of central tubercle or calcification center.

3. Hypocalcemia = pitting type EH; TETANY= due to decreased levels of Ca^{++} in blood, i.e. < 6-8 mg %; e.g. in vit D deficiency, parathyroid deficiency.
4. Birth injuries = neonatal line = due to change in environment; seen in primary teeth and permanent first molars; more common in premature babies and Rh hemolytic birth disease at birth.
5. Local infection / trauma = <u>Turner's tooth</u> = single tooth is involved; esp max 1, 2, 4, 5 and mand 4, 5. Seen as brownish/ yellowish stain or pitting type defect.
6. Flouride = seen by McKay and Black 1916; normal level = 1 ppm;

EH is due to disturbances of ameloblasts during formative stage; and interference with calcification process of matrix;

Grading of fluorosis

- Questionable = white flecks / spotting of enamel
- Mild = white opaque areas
- Moderate / severe = pitting / brownish staining
- Corroded appearance of teeth

C. DENTINOGENESIS IMPERFECTA: aka hereditary opalescent dentin

- Only mesodermal part is affected;
- Type I = DI + OI-esp deciduous teeth affected
- Type II = DI only; ka HOD, both primary/ permanent teeth affected. It is AD trait.
- Type III = DI of Brandy-wine type; multiple pulp exposures are seen in primary teeth; but not in type I, II.
- Color of teeth has unusual transluscent / opalescent hue.
- Enamel lost earlier due to fracture; defective DEJ.; dentin worn off;
- R/G = in type I,II = obliteration of pulp chambers and RCs by continued formation of dentin; in both primary/permanent teeth

- In **type III = shell teeth-**where enamel is normal; dentin is very thin; enormous pulp chambers; roots are very short; dentin tubules are larger dia./ less in number; increased water content of dentin; 60 % above normal; and inorganic content is less than normal dentin; so hardness is decreased which is approx that of cementum.

D. DENTIN DYSPLASIA: aka **rootless teeth**

— Normal enamel; atypical dentin; abnormal pulp morphology;

• Type I = DD ka radicular DD, in both dentitions; abnormal mobility of teeth; premature fall due to rootless;

• Type II = anomalous dysplasia of dentin; ka coronal DD.; affects both dentitions

R/G =

Type I = deciduous= pulp chambers/ RC completely obliterated,

Permanent = crescent shaped ramnants seen in pulp chambers, PA radiolucencies are v. common.

Type II = deciduous = PC obliterated like type I and DI

Permanent = abnormally large coronal pulp chambers ka *thistle-tube* in shape; having radiopaque foci like pulp stones; NO PA RADIOLUCENCIES

H/E = TYPE I = **lava flowing around boulders**; due to repeated attempts to form root structures; dentin is normal but disoriented;

Type II = in deciduous teeth = atubular dentin in root; normal dentin in coronal part

But in permanent teeth = multiple pulp stones; normal coronal dentin.

E. REGIONAL ODONTODYSPLASIA: ka odontogenic imperfecta; **ghost teeth**

- Esp in 1, 2, 3, teeth both U/L
- Due to local vascular deficit;
- Delayed/total failure of eruption
- Defective mineralization

- R/G = marked decrease in radiodensity; pulp chambers are very large , v. thin E/D.
- H/E = marked decreased amount in dentin; widened predentin layer; large areas of interglobular dentin

F. DENTIN HYPOCALCIFICATION = large areas of uncalcified interglobular dentin; softer

G. ERUPTION DISTURBANCES

Natal teeth	At birth
Neonatal teeth	Within 30 days of birth; mainly deciduous mand incisors
Premature eruption	In hyperthyroidism, hyperpituitarism; adrenogenital synd;
Delayed eruption	In rickets; cretinism; cleidocranial dysplasia; hypopituitarism;
Multiple unerupted teeth	Cleidocranial dysplasia
Embedded teeth	Due to lack of eruptive force
Impacted teeth	Due to physical barrier in eruption path, e.g. mand 8 > max 8; also 8 > max 3 > 4,5 > supernumerery teeth
Submerged teeth	Ankylosed deciduous tooth esp mand E; solid sound on percussion

H. COMMON SITES

Dens invaginatus	Max 2
Dens evaginatus	Premolars
Talon's cusp	U/L incisors
Microdontia	Max 2, 8
Taurodontism	Molars

H. Common Sites (*Contd.*)

Supernumerary roots	Mand 3, 4, 5, 8 & max 8
Anodontia	8 > mand 5 > max 5 > max 2
Supernumerary tooth	Max mesiodens; max distomolars
Pseudo-deciduous dentition	Mand incisors
Enamel hypoplasia with nutritional deficiency	1, 2, 6, and tip of 3
Congenital syphilis	Max and mand 1, 2, 6

I. STAGES OF DEFORMITY DEVELOPMENTS

Initiation and proliferation	Missing teeth; supernumerary teeth; fusion; gemination
Histodifferentiation, i.e. structure	Dentinogenesis imperfecta; dentinal dysplasia; shell teeth (type III DI); odontodysplasia, i.e. ghost teeth (dentin related condition)
Morphodifferentiation, i.e. form	Peg laterals; microdontia; macrodontia; dens-in-dente; mulberry molars; talon's cusp
Apposition/ amount	Hypoplasia; AI; intrinsic stains; fluorosis; concrescence;
Hardness	Hypocalcified E and D; interglobular dentin; AI;

In fluorosis = enamel is hypomineralised;

- diff. B/w facial hemihypertrophy, neurofibromatosis/ fibrous dysplasia = teeth size and rate of eruption is increased in facial hemihypertrophy.

J. CLEFT LIP AND PALATE

- Due to failure of mesodermal penetration of and obliteration of ectodermal grooves separating these mesodermal masses, i.e. facial processes.
- Polygenic inheritance, heredity = most common cause
- 1:800, if mother's age is increased;
- unilateral > bilateral; complete > incomplete in incidence.
- CL /CP = M > F; CL = L > R (3:1); Isolated CP = F > M;
- Associated development defects are more common with isolated CP than CL with /without CP (50% vs 20%).
- Rule of 10's = 10 gm % Hb; 10 lbs wt.; 10 weeks age; 10,000 WBCs = **lip repair**

DEVELOPMENTAL CYSTS

Dev. by entrapped epith. along fusion lines ka fissural /inclusion cysts; these are <u>true cysts</u>.

Median ant max cyst	Most common type of max dev cyst; aka nasopalatine duct/ incisive canal cyst;
Median alveolar cyst	Primordial, odontogenic, From supernum. mesiodens tooth bud; heart shaped on R/G; between roots of max centrals in midline;
Median palatal cyst	From epith b/w the line of fusion of palatal processes of maxilla, seen in PM and molar region on R/G.
Globullomaxillary cyst	From epith b/w max. pr. and MNP; i.e. b/w max 2 and 3; b/w premax and max; teeth are <u>vital</u>
Median mand cyst	v. rare, pulp <u>vital</u>; R/G= unilocular, well circumscribed

Nasoalveolar/ nasolabial/ Klestadt's cyst	Arise at the junction of globular process & LNP and max. process; From lower ant part of nasolacrimal duct; it is not present in bone but in soft tissues; in b/w max 2 and 3 area; Swelling is near alar attachment; Superficial erosion of outer surface of maxilla;
Palatal cysts of neonates	1. **Bohn's nodules** = at junction of hard & soft palates; dev. from palatal salivary glands 2. **Epstein's pearls** = along median raphe of hard palate; dev. from entrapped epith. remnants 3. Dental lamina cysts of newborns = on alveolar ridge; dev. from dental lamina / odontogenic; most common along median raphe
Thyroglossal tract cysts	B/w F. ceacum and thyroid glands; arise from remnants of this tract; from the cells originating from embryonic pharyngeal floor
Branchial cleft cyst	Aka benign cervical lymphoepithelial cyst; Occurs on lateral aspect of neck; at ant border of SCM m; Arises from remnants of branchial arches or pharyngeal pouches
Dermoid cyst	From embryonic germinal epithelium during closure of mand and hyoid branchial arches; lie in floor of mouth, submax, sublingual regions Bulging in the floor of mouth = if cyst is b/w geniohyoid and oral mm, i.e. above the GH muscle, Bulging in submental area = if cyst lies below GH m i.e. b/w GH and MH ms.

BLOOD PATHOLOGIES

Pernicious anemia/ Addison's disease/ Biermer's anemia	• Deficiency of *intrinsic factor*, due to atrophy of gastric mucosa. • intrinsic factor helps absorption of Vit. B_{12}, the *extrinsic factor* from intestine; vit B_{12} is erythrocyte-maturing factor and is present in beef, liver, milk and dairy products. • C/F = *triad* = generalised weakness; sore painful tongue; numbness/ tingling of extremities. • Nervous system involved = due to degeneration of posterior and lateral tracts of spinal cord, of myelin sheath and loss of nerve fibres. • Tongue = beefy red; gradual atrophy of papillae = bald tongue ks Hunter's/ Moeller's glossitis • Oral mucosa = intolerant to dentures • Lab diagnosis = macrocytosis = chief C/F • **Howell- Jolly bodies** and **Cabot's ring** of RBCs abnormalities in advanced stages. • Magaloblasts increased in numbers, decreased RBCs, WBCs, Hb • Achlorhydria/ lack of gastric HCl = so pH of gastric contents is high due to gastric mucosa atrophy and decreased number of parietal cells; gastric cancer in these patients. • Decreased Argentaffin cells in stomach and intestine
Sprue/idiopathic steatorrhoea/ celiac disease	1. Is a malabsorption syndrome; glossitis & diarrhoea 2. Esp in patients on diet deficient in vit B_{12} or folic acid. 3. Due to intolerance of gluten wheat/rye flour 4. Aka Gee- Herter dis. = when occurs in children

Blood Pathologies (*Contd.*)

	5. Steatorrhoea occurs due to fibrocystic dis.of pancreas and decrease in pancreatic enzyme secretions. 6. C/F = excess loss of fats and calcium in stools and so occasional TETANY; nervous irritation/numbness but no spinal cord involvement.; brownish skin pigmentations 7. O/F = glossitis = atrophy of filiform papillae 8. Lab = macrocytic anemia; leucopenia
Aplastic anemia	• Pancytopenia = decreased RBC, WBC, Platelets, HCt • 2 types = primary = unknown etiology; bad prognosis • **fanconi's synd** = familial/ congenital AA; ass. with congenital deformities and olive-brown skin pigmentations. • Secondary AA = known causes; better prognosis, • C/F = numbness of extremities, petechiae due to less platelets; infections due to less WBCs
Thalassemia Cooley's anemia/ erythroblastic anemia	1. Occurs below 2 yeas age; 2. Alpha-thalassemia = deficient synthesis of alpha chain 3. Beta-thalassemia = deficient synthesis of beta chain 4. Thalassemia-minor / thalassemia Trait = in heterozygotes 5. Thalassemia major = severe form; homozygotes; 6. Hemoglobin-H dis. = mild form **7. Hb-Bart's disease** = with hydrops fetalis-infants are stillborn.

Blood Pathologies (*Contd.*)

	8. C/F =mongoloid face, due to prominent cheek bones and depressed nasal bridge; 9. O/F = prominent premaxilla; 10. Lab = **hypochromic microcytic anemia**; contains Hb- F (fetal), RBCs seen as target cells; p.o. safety pin cells and normoblasts i.e. nucleated RBCs; increased hemosiderosis and blocked iron use; 11. R/G = **crew- cut / hair on end appearance** of skull surface; 12. IOPA = salt & pepper effect in jaws due to mild osteoporosis; thinning of lamina dura;
Sickle cell anemia	Hb-S is produced due to substitution of valine for glutamine at 6 th position of beta- globin chain; sickle shaped cells. **Sickle cell trait** = if heterozygous; 40 % Hb-S present;C/F = packing of RBCs in peripheral vessels leading to local tissue anoxia; **Sickle cell crisis** = during GA; due to decreased oxygenation of blood. O/F = generalised osteoporosis; loss of bony trabeculae esp in alveolar bone; no change in lamina dura or PDL; R/G = **hair on end appearance** on skull; tower-shaped skull; generalised osteoporosis; thin cortices; enlarged medullary cavities;
Erythroblastosis fetalis	Congenital hemolytic anemia due to Rh incompatibility; strongest Rh- antigen is D-antigen; occurs when father is Rh + ve and mother is Rh – ve, so kid is Rh – ve, so antibodies are produced; First pregnancy is uneventful. Rh-ve mothers are given anti-D gamma globulins to prevent immunisation, i.e. RHOGAM.

Blood Pathologies (*Contd.*)

	C/F = + ve direct coomb's test on cord blood; O/F = green/ blue / brown discolor of teeth = due to bilirubin; it affects only deciduous teeth; stains are intrinsic; Enamel hypoplasia= a ring like defect ka **Rh-hump** occurs.
Iron deficiency anemia/ Plummer – Vinson synd	Predisposing factor = oral cancer and of upper GIT C/F = smooth red painful tongue = atrophy of filiform papillae Dysphagia due to oesophageal stricture/web. Mucous memb atrophy due to iron deficiency. Lab = microcytic, hypochromic anemia; no megaloblasts in sternal marrow; decreased Hb, RBC, serum Fe^{++}, Absence of free radical in stomach. Achlorhydria is the cause of faulty absorption, as Fe^{3+} cannot change to Fe^{2+} then. Confirmatory test = no reticulocyte response to vit B_{12} administration.
Polycythemia	Primary / Osler's dis / Vaquez disease Or poly. Rubra vera = C/F = skin blushing due to capillary engorgements, splenomegaly; cyanosis of digits/ tongue/gingiva = due to amount of reduced Hb > 5 gm%. **Treatment** = phenylhydrazine = for destruction of blood N2-mustard, P 32, X-rays = to interfere with blood formation
Leukopenia	Decreased WBC esp granulocytes;
Agranulocytosis/ neutropenia	Most common cause = drugs Basic defect is in arrest of cell maturation C/F = most imp = p.o. infections esp in oral cavity; necrotising ragged ulcers; **little/no**

Blood Pathologies (*Contd.*)

	inflammatory cell infiltration in lesions; all oral surgeries are C/I. H/E = rapid gingival necrosis and destruction of tissues. Lab = WBC < 2000, complete absence of PMN/granulocytes,
Cyclic neutropenia	Cyclic decrease in PMN neutrophils; Rapid gingivitis, loss of superficial alv bone; ka prepubertal peridontitis in children; **Cycle commonly occurs after every 3 weeks**. In blood, neutrophil decrease is compensated by increased monocytes and lymphocytes. Splenectomy is beneficial treatment.
Chediak-Higashi synd	Fatal in early life; oculocutaneous albinism Sometimes ass. with malignant lymphomas; Ulcers, PDL breakdown due to defective WBCs, Lab = giant abnormal granules in peripheral leucocytes, a hallmark of synd, they are abnormal lysosomes.
Infectious mononucleosis/ glandular fever	Ka **kissing dis**; caused by EB virus (which also causes burkitt's lymphoma, nasopharyngeal ca., lymphoblastic leukemia) C/F = cervical/ axilla/ groin LAP; pin point petechiae at the junction of hard and soft palate. Lab = atypical lymphocytes, Abs to EBV; increased heterophil titre to 1: 4096 (N = 1: 8), it is ka Paul-Bunnel test. Increased WBC esp lymphocytosis; patient has > 50 % lymphocytosis, during acute phase = pt has normal ESR.

Leukemia: 3 types

- Myeloid/ myelocytic L = involves granulocytes
- Lymphoid / lymphocytic L = involves lymphocytes
- Monocytic = involves monocytes

Etiology =

1. Polyoma Virus = in animals
2. **EBV** = in humans
3. Chromosomal = *philadelphia* chr.= CMyL. It is translocation from chr 22 to chr 9
4. Downs synd = acute leukemia,
5. Acute is more common in children than adults.
6. Acute L of adults is mostly of monocytic type
7. LAP is common in CLL, but not in CML.
8. Subleukemic L = in it, WBC count is normal or subnormal, and there are no immmature WBCs present.
9. Acute L = LAP is the first sign; haemorrhages due to decreased platelets; terminal infections due to crowding out of myeloid tissues; WBCs > 100,000 / mm ^{3}
10. Stem cell L = leukemic cells are highly undifferentiated; most difficult to diagnose;
11. Chronic L = WBCs > 500,000 / mm^3
12. Oral C/F = most common in A Mo L; gingival haemmorhage is due to ulceration of sulcus epithelium and necrosis of underlying tissues.
13. No inflammatory response = as WBCs are disturbed.

SPECIAL FEATURES

AMoL	Gingival enlargement; oral lesions
ALL	CNS involvement; mostly in children
CML	is associated with **philadelphia chromosome** (T 22,9 chr), (90%); Spleen enlargement

CLL	caused by **RNA type-C tumor virus**; Liver enlargement
AML	**Worst prognosis**
ALL	Commonest in childhood; least likely to produce oral lesions
Chloroma	L involving bone marrow of orbit and skull.

HEAMOPHILIA-A = is most common type of H.

• 50-70 % level or at least 30 % level in blood of factor VIII is required in hemophiliac-A patient = for dental extraction or surgery.

• Hemo-A patients are given factor VIII replacement therapy with cryoprecipitates, which is prepared from fresh plasma

• **Tranexamic acid** = antifibrolytic agent = may help in m/m of bleeding. It reduces the amount of AHF that needs to be given, but it is not a substitute for AHF.

• Factor VIII deficiency is a C/I for inferior alveolar n. block = because bleeding in deeper tissues leads to asphyxia.

• Factor VIII def. causes bleeding, which characteristically ceases within minutes, to recur after an hour or so, and then persists.

In pernicious anemia = decreased argentaffin cells in stomach and intestine.

Most striking lesion of oral m.m in vit.B complex def. = pellagra (niacin def.)

Skin pigmentations

- Sprue = brownish
- Aplastic anemia = olive-brown skin pigmentations.
- Hyperparathyroidism
- Neurofibromatosis

PLATELETS DISEASES

Purpura =

- **Non-thrombocytopenic purpura** = not htrough platelets but defect of capillaries;eg increased permeability, fragility
- **Thrombocytopenic purpura** = decreased number of platelets;
- **Primary thrombocytopenic purpura** = aka **Werlhoff's dis**; of unknown etiology, is an autoimmune disease; antiplatelet globulin/ antibodies to platelets in blood; spleen is not palpable; severe and profuse gingival bleeding, so any oral surgery is C/I untill controlled; platelets are < 60,000 / mm 3; increased BT; + ve tourniquet / Hess's test;
- Cessation of bleeding depends on physical blockade of severed capillaries by platelets which depends on number of platelets; treatment = splenectomy.
- Thrombotic TP = transient neurologic dysfunction; widespread microthrombi in body; occlusive subintimal deposits at arteriocapillary junctions

Aldrich's synd =

- In males only; XR,
- Infections are due to Ab-deficiency, i.e. poor Ab response to polysaccharide antigen;
- Serum IgM decreased; so patient is not able to form Abs to polysach.-containing organisms, i.e. *Pneumococci, H. influenzae,* coliform bacilli;
- Lymphoreticular malignant neoplasms / malignant lymphomas

Thrombocytasthenia = a QUALITATIVE defect in platelets

- Familial = excessive bleeding; onset of menarche in females is very critical.
- Treatment = epsilon–ACA to control post-op. bleeding.

Thrombocytopathic purpura = aka thrombocytopathia

1. Platelet count is NORMAL.
2. Storage pool dis = deficient platelet adenine nucleotide

3. Portsmouth synd = abnormal collagen induced aggregation
4. Bernard-Soulier synd = abnormal response to fibrinogen

Thrombocythemia = thrombocytosis

- Increased number of circulating platelets,
- Treatment = radioactive phosphorus P^{32}

HEMOPHILIA: **bleeder's dis** / dis of **Hapsburgs**

- X-recessive, only in males
- Hemophilia A = Most common; due to AHG (Factor VIII) deficiency.
- Hemophilia B = Christmas disease, due to PTC (Factor IX) DEFICIENCY
- **Hemophilia C** = due to PTA (Factor XI) deficiency,
- In hemo-A, i.e. classic hemo – only clot – promoting factor is absent, so prothrombin does not change to thrombin.
- C/F = gingival hemorrhages, **mandibular pseudotumors** – due to subperiosteal bleeding and reactive bone formation.
- Tooth extraction = massive bleeding, so it should be done with rubber bands/ pressure necrosis,
- Lab = increased CT, normal BT, PT,
- Treatment = pre-op transfusion of whole blood and AHG conc.
- Pre-op = factor VIII conc.
- Post-op = epsilon ACA

Von-willebrand's dis = aka pseudohemophilia

1. Only BT is prolonged–excessive bleeding
2. Autosomal dominant; more in females
3. Classic hemophilia is caused by a deficiency of one of the 3 components of factor 8, but classic Von-Willebrand's dis is due to decrease in all the 3 components of factor 8.

Parahemophilia

- Is due to deficiency of factor V, i.e. proaccelerin, which causes prothrombin to thrombin.

Afibrinogenemia/hypofibrinogenopenia

- No fibrinogen/factor I in blood = so blood cannot clot even after adding thrombin.
- Congenital type = inability to synthesise fibrinogen; complete absence of fibrinogen
- Acquired type = defective fibrinogen formation.
- CT and PT are INFINITE. ESR is zero.

Dysfibrinogenemia

1. Fibrinogen detroit = in it, arginine replaces serine.
2. Fibrinogen philadelphia = in it, abnormal protein is catabolised at an increased rate.
3. Fibrinogen is normal in amount, but defective in structure and coagulability.

Factor XIII deficiency

Pt has severe post- surgical bleeding, which are delayed for 24–36 hours.

. Factor XIII helps in stabilising the fibrin framework.

Macroglobulinemia = of Waldenstrom

- Is a plasma cell dyscrasia so that increased proliferation of B-cells results in production of large amount of M-type of Ig M globulins characteristic of disease.

Cryoglobulinemia = i.e. globulins which precipitates on exposure to cold and redissolves on body temp.; seen in collagen-dis; lymphomas.

TUMORS OF ORAL CAVITY

Papilloma	Cauliflower like surface; papilloma virus is the cause. Pebbly surface = is in **Cowden's syndrome;** Is considered the cutaneous marker of breast cancer
Keratoacanthoma	Self-healing carcinoma; occurs mainly on exposed skin;
Nevi	Small nevi = 1–5 cm; garment nevi > 10 cm in size Acquired nevi are v.v common; appear at about 8 months age; Intradermal nevi = one of the most common lesions of skin; Compound nevi = i.e. intradermal + junctional nevi Spindle cell/ epitheloid nevi = esp in children; is histologically malignant; i.e. resembles malignant melanoma. Blue nevi = is a true mesodermal structure; In oral cavity = acquired N except Spindle cell/ epitheloid nevi occur H/E = nevus cells are derived from neural crests; arranged in alveolar patterns ka **theques,** I/D nevus = cells are within CT; separated from epithelium by a well defined band of CT. Junctional nevi = cells blend with the epithelium; epthelial cells are seen growing down in the CT ka OBTROPFUNG / dropping off EFFECT; undergoes malignant transformation; Congenital N = greater risk of malignant transformation B-K mole synd = large pigmented nevi and high risk of development of melanomas.

Tumors of Oral Cavity (*Contd.*)

Leukoplakia	Premalignant; hyperkeratotic; transforms to epidermoid ca., Vit A deficiency = causes metaplasia/ keratinisation of epith. Vit B def = causes alteration of oxidation pattern of epithelium; **Pipe smoker's palate** = aka stomatitis nicotina = partially occluded orifices of accessory palatal salivary glands ducts. *Hyperorthokeratosis* = is an abnormal increase in thickness of orthokeratin layer or stratum corneum at particular locations *Hyperparakeratosis* = i.e. nuclei/nuclear re-mnants persist *Acanthosis* = abnormal thickening of spinous layer i.e. prickle cell layer *Dyskaryosis* = nuclear atypism, e.g. giant cells Poikilocarynosis = division of nuclei without division of cytoplasm *Malignant dysplasia* = aka dyskeratosis *Benign dyskeratosis* = e.g. in Darrier's dis, molluscum contagiosum **Carcinoma-in - situ** = intraepithelial ca., top to bottom basilar hyperplasia is seen D/D = lichen planus is the most imp. lesion
Leukodema	Mostly seen on buccal mucosa along posterior occlusal plane Intracellular oedema of spinous or malphigian layer
Intraepithelial ca. Aka carcinoma–in situ	It is laterally spreading, intraepithelial type of ca., with no invasive potential at this stage; **Bowen's dis** = esp in patients on *Arsenic* therapy H/E = individual cell keratinisation is very rare, which is the **hallmark of transfor-**

Tumors of Oral Cavity (*Contd.*)

	mation of Intraepithelial ca. in invasive ca. All the changes occur within the surface epithelium, which remains confined to basement membrane.
Erythroplakia (of Queyrat)	Red color is due to = CT pegs extend very high into the epithelium, carrying capillary loops with them.
Oral submucous fibrosis	Precancerous condition; C/F = burning sensation of mouth with spices; Fibrotic bands; stiffening of mucosa; trismus; H/E = oral epithelium is extremely atrophic; with loss of rete-pegs Treatment = inj. Placentrix; vit A and E
Basal cell ca. Or rodent ulcer	Occur on skin only; does not arise from OMM; **never seen in oral cavity**; causes direct invasion and erosion of tissues; No tendency of metastasis; aka benign ca., C/F = ulcer has smooth rolled out margins representing tumor cells spreading laterally beneath the skin. Mostly seen in MID THIRD OF FACE Multiple BCC = in "jaw cyst–bifid rib–basal cell nevus synd"
Squamous cell ca./epidermoid ca.	Most common malignant tumor of oral cavity; Seen in **Plummer –Vinsom synd**; Various viruses are also assoc. = 1. EBV = infectious mononucleosis; Burkitt's tumor; nasopharyngeal ca. 2. CMV = cytomegalic inclusion disease, Kaposi sarcoma 3. HSV = herpes simplex infection 4. VZV = chicken pox; herpes zoster; shingles; not assoc. with any human malignant ca.

Tumors of Oral Cavity (*Contd.*)

	5. HSV II = ca. of uterine cervix H/E = rapid metastatic spread; blood stream metastasis is ucommon,
Ca. of lip	Begins on vermillion border of lips; mostly on lower lip;
Ca. of tongue	Esp in syphilis; lesions develop on the lateral border/ ventral surface of tongue; lesions of base have poorest prognosis;
Verrucous ca.	H/E is very deceptive; downgrowth of epithelium in CT without evidence of invasion; Cleft like spaces lined by a thick layer of parakeratin seen = as a hallmark of this lesion
Malignant melanoma	3rd most common cancer of skin; (SCC>BCC). Is a neoplasm of epidermal melanocytes; **Sunlight is** an imp etiological factor 2 phases of growth of melanomas occur = 1. Radial = initial phase, neoplastic cells confined to epidermis; 2. Vertical = metastasis is possible in this phase. Types = 3 1. Superficial spreading = most common; radial growth phase; aka premalignant melanosis. H/E = intraepithelial phase, i.e. radial growth pattern = the melanocytes are in PAGETOID MANNER; In CT = FLORID manner; 2. Nodular melanoma = exists only in vertical growth pattern. Exists in CT only; malignant 3. Lentigo maligna melanoma = not seen on OMM; radial growth pattern; aka **melanotic freckle of Hutchinson**. It occurs as a MACULAR lesion **on malar skin** of

Tumors of Oral Cavity (*Contd.*)

	middle aged. Increase in atypical melanocytes within basal epithelial layer; ♦ Significantly, focal pigmentation occurs months before the appearance of clinical neoplasm – so any increase in size / pigmentation should be viewed seriously. ♦ If occur on BANS areas = if > 0.75 mm, the prognosis is poor and has a great tendency of metastasis. ♦ Depth of invasion suggest prognosis = so superficial spreading and nodular have poor prognosis than lentigo maligna.
Fibroma	Most common benign CT tumor in oral cavity
Peripheral ossifying/ cementifying/ odontogenic fibroma	Derived from PDL; Occur anterior to molars; on the gingiva, papilla; more common in children/young appears to originate from I/D adults. H/E = very high degree of cellularity, esp fibroblasts may cause superficial erosion of bone.
Central ossifying fibroma	In mandible/ black females; teeth displacement H/E = **Chinese-letter pattern** of bony trabeculae, as in fibrous dysplasia of bone. R/G = lesion is well demarcated from the surroundings
Peripheral giant cell granuloma/ osteoclastoma	Arises due to trauma esp extraction; Always on gingiva/alv. Process = anterior to molars Origin from PDL or mucoperiosteum; R/G = shows **peripheral cuffing** of bone due to superficial erosion.

Tumors of Oral Cavity (*Contd.*)

Central giant cell granuloma	Single bone lesion; reported only in jaws; Involves anterior part of the jaws; may cross the midline; Treatment = with **radiation is C/I**.
Aneurysmal bone cyst	In young; blood soaked spongy tissue; R/G = **honey-comb / soap bubble** appearance; eccentrically ballooned; ♦ There remains the circulatory connection with damaged blood vessels; but not in GC granuloma
Verucous xanthoma/ histiocytosis Y	H/E = severe parakeratotic plugging; Large, swollen, *foam cells/xanthoma cells,* i.e. histiocytes = they do not extend into the dermis beneath the epithelial pegs and are confined to papilla only.
Hemangioma	Not a true neoplasm; central type is seen as HONEYCOMB and SUN–BURST APPEARANCE on R/G;
Hamartoma	An abnormal proliferation of tissues of structures native to that place
Rendu-Osler Weber's disease	Hereditary hemorrhagic telengiectasia; spider-like telengiectasia; due to repeated hemorrhages; ♦ Earliest sign of this dis = epistaxis and bleeding from oral cavity which is difficult to control. ♦ H/E = defects in small blood vessels; weak perivascular supporting tissues
Sturge-Weber synd/encephalo-trigeminal angiomatosis	1. Venous angiomas of leptomeninges over cerebral cortex + ipsilateral angiomatous lesions of face, skull, jaws, etc.; 2. Dermal capillary–venous angiomas, i.e. port-wine nevi present **confined to skin areas supplied by 5th nerve**

Tumors of Oral Cavity (*Contd.*)

	3. Intracranial convolutional calcifications ka RAIL ROAD CALCIFICATIONS 4. Neurologic manifestations = convulsive disorders and spastic hemiplegia
Lymphangiomas	Most common on *tongue* esp anterior-dorsal part; In less than 10 years of age child; Macroglossia and irregular nodularity of the surface
Oral focal mucinosis	Dev. due to fibroblastic overproduction of hyaluronic acid and it lacks reticulin network
Chondroma	Benign central tumor; seldom develops in MEMBRANOUS BONES; but can develop in Mx/Md which have vestigial C-where it can develop; 1. Mx = malar process near molars and pre-maxillary area have vestigial C. Anterior part of Mx is the most common site – as vestigial C. rests are present esp in midline lingual to / between central incisors; 2. Md. = mental region, coronoid and condyle have vestigial C. The most common site is posterior to cuspids – involving body of mandible or coronoid/condyle 3. It is resistant to RADIATIONS
Codman's tumor	Aka benign chondroblastoma; is MNGC (multinucleated giant cells) lesion
Osteoma	Multiple osteomas are seen in GARDNER'S SYND
Chondromyxoid fibroma	PAIN is an outstanding feature

Tumors of Oral Cavity (*Contd.*)

Osteoid osteoma	R/G = pathognomic picture as – small ovoid / round R/L areas – surrounded by a rim of sclerotic bone
Benign osteoblastoma	Painful; most common in *vertebral* column
Torus mandibularis	Mostly in *bicuspid area* on lingual side; above the mylohyoid line
Multiple exostosis	On buccal surface of maxilla below the mucobuccal folds in molar region

MALIGNANT TUMORS

Fibrosarcoma	Sarcomas differ from malignant epithelium neoplasms by their typical occurrence in relatively *young persons* and their greater tendency to **metastasize through the blood stream** rather through lymphatics.
Hemangio-pericytoma	1. Profuse proliferation of occult capillaries 2. Pericytes of Zimmerman are found pre-dominantly – a cell with contractile pro-perties but no myofibrils, resemble *glomus* tumor cells 3. Cells show a characteristic tendency for concentric layering about the capillaries
Multiple idiopathic hemorrhagic sarcoma of KAPOSI	Is an infectious granuloma or RE hyperplasia; Initial lesion is polyvasculitis; Decrease T-cells Caused by CMV; also found in AIDS
Ewing's sarcoma/ round cell sarcoma	From RE cells; primary destructive lesion of bone; mostly in children; Rapid onset of jaw swelling; pain; facial neuralgias;

Malignant Tumors (*Contd.*)

Or endothelial myeloma	R/G = ONION-SKIN APPEARANCE – due to formation of layers of new sub- periosteal bone. ♦ Osteophyte formation – gives SUN-RAY APPEARANCE of osteosarcoma ♦ H/E = extremely cellular; ABSENT MNGCs; ♦ Cells contain glycogen (which is absent in reticulum cell sarcoma)
Chondrosarcoma	Invasive, destructive, metastasizes early Treatment = wide excision should be done = *surgical intervention* often stimulates the growth rate and increases tendency to metastasize.
Osteosarcoma	1. With definite history of trauma 2. Also appears in bones affected by paget's disease 3. With X- rays = it may undergo malignant transformation 4. R/G = SUN-RAY APPEARANCE = in sclerosing form 5. A **symmetrically widened PDL** space around one or more teeth 6. Metastasis is more common to **lungs**.
Malignant lymphoma	Derived from basic cells of lymphoid tissues; Occurs in an essentially homogenous population of single cell type ♦ Lymphomas and leukemias of lymphocytes and histiocytes are identical.
Non-Hodgkin's lymphomas; NHL	Involves both lymph nodes and lymphoid organs as well as extranodal organs and tissues; esp of head and neck areas Extranodal involvement is in > 60 yrs age Waldeyer's ring is the most common site

Malignant Tumors (*Contd.*)

	Nodular type = of B –cells origin Diffuse type = mostly B-cells origin; but T-cells also
Burkitt's lymphoma/ African jaw tumor	1. EBV is the cause 2. Non-Hodgkin's lymphoma; B-cell origin 3. Endemic form = mainly in children of 2 – 14 yrs age; mainly involves extranodal tissues (as cp. To NHL) 4. Non-endemic form = involves LNs and lymphoid tissues esp bone marrow; visceral involvement is more common 5. H/E = macrophages scattered through out the tumor = STARRY-SKY EFFECT
Hodgkin's lymphomas	Primarily, a disease of LNs; mainly LNs & lymphoid organs; esp cervical LNs are involved initially; BIMODAL AGE OCCURRENCE = incidence peak in young adults and 5th decade; H/E = multinucleated REED-STERNBEG CELLS (RS cells) = are of lymphocytic origin RS cells in nodular sclerosis are aka LACUNAR CELLS *4 types* = lymphocytic predominant; nodular sclerosis; mixed cellularity; lymphocytic depletion types ♦ LP = best prognosis ♦ LD = worst prognosis ♦ MC = more in males ♦ NS = more in females ♦ NS and LP = on one side of diaphragm ♦ Diagnosed by = Gordon's biologic test
Multiple myeloma/ plasmacytoma	Multicentric/ multiple bone origin; arise from cells of bone marrow; Arise in ramus, angle, molar area of mandible = which are most active hematopoietic areas

Malignant Tumors (*Contd.*)

	R/G = SHARPLY PUNCHED OUT LESIONS ♦ **Bence-Jones proteins in** urine, which coagulate at 40–60° C, and disappear on boiling. ♦ Reversal of serum albumin – globulin ratio ♦ Increase in total serum proteins = to 8–16 gm% ♦ H/E = plasma cells with CART WHEEL/ CHECKERBOARD PATTERN ♦ **Russell bodies** = common as in chronic inflammatory lesions

TUMORS OF MUSCLE ORIGINS

Leiomyoma	Benign; form smooth ms; In oral cavity = smooth ms are found in walls of blood vessels & circumvallate papillae of tongue; so it is found in posterior part of tongue mostly
Rhabdomyoma	From striated ms; mostly tongue and floor of mouth
Granular cell myoblastoma/ myoblastic myoma	Most common on tongue; arises from **Schwann cells;** tumors cells get stained intensely with antiserum to S-100 protein S-100 protein is mainly found outside CNS only in Schwann cells; stellate cells of ganglia; also in schwannomas and neurofibromas
Leiomyosarcomas	Malignant tumor of smooth ms; on cheek and floor of mouth
Rhabdo-myosarcoma	Pleomorphic rhabdomyosarcomas have RACQUET CELLS, i.e. large cells with nuclei situated often in an expanded end of the cell Alveolar rhabdomyosarcomas-epithelial like

Tumors of Muscle Origins (*Contd.*)

	cells dropping off from collagen trabeculae; cells floating in alveolar space are common.
Traumatic/ amputation neuroma	1. Derived mainly from perineurium 2. Generally occur near the mental foramen 3. Exuberant attempt to **repair of a damaged nerve trunk** 4. Limited to areas bordering mucocutaneous junctions, predominantly on face
Multiple endocrine neoplasia; MEN syndromes	MEN I = **Weiner's syndrome**; tumors (of pituitary/parathyroid/adrenal cortex and pancreatic islets of Langerhans) + peptic ulcers + gastric hypersecretions MEN II = Sipple's syndrome **IIa** = no pancreas tumors and no peptic ulcer; but parathyroid hyperplasia + pheochromocytomas of adrenal medulla + medullary ca. of thyroid MEN III = **IIb;** mucocutaneous neuromas; pheochromocytomas of adrenal medulla + medullary ca. of thyroid; marfanoid habitus; hypertrophied corneal nerves, etc. ♦ More common components of MEN III is = NEUROMAS; bumpy lips ♦ medullary ca. of thyroid = can metastasize and cause death
Melanotic neuroectodermal tumor of infancy	Aka pigmented/ melanotic ameloblastoma; Occurs < 6 mos age. High urinary excretion of vanillyl mandellic acid (VMA), supports NCC origin
Metastatic tumors of jaws	Mostly in mandible; in molar area as it contains rich deposits of hematopoietic tissues. Plexus of vertebral (Batson's plexus) Vs is dissemination blood –route

Tumors of Muscle Origins (*Contd.*)

•	Osteoblastic lesions are associated with ca. Prostate, breast and lungs Ca. Thyroid was the most common metastatic tumor of the jaws; but now is **ca. of lungs** has increased %age.
Juxtaoral organ of CHIEVITZ	Is cluster of nests of sq. epith. cells; associated with myelinated Ns; Have neuro-endocrine receptor functions

Neurofibroma / fibroma molluscum	**Neurolemmoma**
H/E = no capsule; Neurites present	Capsulated; No neurites
	♦ Antoni type A tissues = cells with elongated or spindle shaped nuclei, aligned in a palisade manner; intracellular fibres arranged in parallel fashion ♦ Antoni type A tissues = no palisade pattern. Microcysts due to intracellular oedema ♦ Verocay bodies present
Arise from Schwann cells, fibroblasts, perineurial cells	Form Schwann cells
Multiple nodules	Soft tissue lesion is single nodule
Axillary freckling; hirsutism; macroglossia	
Café-au-lait spots; melanin pigmentation	

Neurofibroma / fibroma molluscum	Neurolemmoma
Central lesion esp in mandible; associated with mandibular nerve	Central lesion = considerable destruction of bone; cortices expansion
R/G = fusiform enlargement of n.and canal	
May undergo malignant transformation after several surgical tempering	Does not undergo malignant transformation

CODMAN'S triangle seen in occlusal R/G, a triangle of new bone at the Junction of subperiosteal sheet of bone with old cortex.

Telengiectasia also seen in:	Solutions for cryotherapy, etc.	PDL widening is seen in =	Bence-Jones proteins in
Scleroderma	CO_2 snow = – 78° C	Osteosarcoma	Multiple myeloma
CREST synd	Liquid N_2 = – 180° C	Scleroderma	Leukemia
Sarcoid diseases	Sclerosing agents = sodium morrhuate or psylliate	Acrosclerosis	Polycythemia
Lupus erythematosis			

WIDE SPREAD SCLEROSIS OF BONES

1. Osteopetrosis
2. Paget's dis

3. Progressive diaphyseal dysplasia
4. Generalised cortical hyperostosis

BLUE SCLERA: in MOORE, i.e.

1. Marfan's synd
2. Osteogenesis imperfecta
3. Osteopetrosis
4. Fetal Rickets
5. Ehler's Danlos synd

INCREASED ALK. P ase: in

1. Caffey's dis
2. Paget's dis
3. Fibrous dysplasia

TUMORS OF SALIVARY GLANDS

These are more common in hard palate than soft palate.

Pleomorphic adenoma/ mixed tumor	Mostly in parotid; **most common salivary gland tumor;** Originates by myoepithelial and reserve cells of intercalated ducts Myoepithelial cells = give morphological diversity: Reserve cells = give ductal + myoepithelial cells Not fixed to underlying tissues. H/E = Always encapsulated; loose myxoid material is a predominant feature.
Warthin's tumor/ papillary cystadenoma lymphomatosum	Monomorphic; exclusively in parotid gland; Intra oral accessory glands are rarely affected Cyst formation is there.

Tumors of Salivary Glands (*Contd.*)

Basal cell adenoma	Arise from intercalated duct / reserve cells; mostly in parotid
Canalicular adenoma	Arise from intraoral accessory glands; in upper lip mainly; H/E = strands or cords of epith. Cells arranged in DOUBLE ROW, showing a PARTY WALL effect.
Oxyphilic adenoma/ oncocytoma	Oncocytes are choked with **mitochondria;** Rare; mainly in parotid
Mikulicz's dis/ benign lymphoepithelial lesion	Has both inflammatory and neoplastic features; Involves **3 glands** = parotid + submax.+ lacrimal H/E = orderly lymphocytic infiltration of salivary gland tissue destroying/replacing acini. Presence of <u>epi-myoepithelial islands</u>
Mikulicz's syndrome	Salivary glands enlarged + lymph nodes enlarged
Sjogren's synd/ Sicca synd	**Triad** = dry eyes (keratoconjuctivitis sicca) + dry mouth (xerostomia) + Rh. Arthritis **Sicca complex/ primary Sjogren's synd** = dry eyes + dry mouth (no Rh. Arthritis) **Secondary Sjogren's synd** = also SLE; polyarteritis nodosa; polymyositis; scleroderma + Rh. Arthritis Etio = autoimmune dis; associated with HLA system esp HLA-DR3 and DR4; most common in females > 40 yrs (M:F = 1: 10) C/F = **"cracked-sound"** on eating biscuits Lab = elevated levels of IgA/K/Na in saliva; polyclonal hyperglobulinemia; cryoglobulins; SSa and SSb antibodies **antisalivary duct antibodies :** 3 times more common in sec.

Tumors of Salivary Glands (*Contd.*)

	than primary syndrome R/G = CHERRY BLOSSOM/BRANCHLESS FRUIT LADEN TREE appearance on sialogram.
Adenoid cystic ca./ cylindroma	Malignant; mostly on palatal mucosa H/E = mucoid material produces a typical cribriform, honey comb or Swiss cheese pattern Spread of tumor cells always along the perineurial spaces/ sheath
Acinic cell ca./ adeno ca.	Most common malignant SG tumor arise from cells of terminal SG ducts Shows acinar cells differentiation, i.e. duct formation Hematogenous metastasis to bones + lungs is common
Mucoepidermoid ca.	Most common malignant SG tumor of **children;** metastasises also Has both mucus secreting and epidermoid type cells Often develop cysts and may resemble **mucocele.**
Central Mucoepidermoid ca. Of jaws	Esp. in molar-premolar region; does not extend anteriorly beyond the premolar area; Resembles **dentigerous cyst** R/G and C/E.
Clear cell ca.	Arise from semi-pleuripotential intercalated duct cells or from myoepithelial cells; mainly in parotid Ka epithelial-myoepithelial Ca. of intercalated duct origin; aka **Donath-Seifert tumor**
Necrotizing sialometaplasia	By local ischemia and acinar coagulation necrosis. Sq. metaplasia occurs in SG ducts when blood supply is compromised

Tumors of Salivary Glands (*Contd.*)

	Mostly occurs on **palate** as ulceration; H/E = preserved lobulated architecture despite necrosis

CYSTS

Primordial cyst	Dev. By cystic degeneration and liquefaction of <u>stellate reticulum</u> in an enamel organ before formation of any calcified tissues; ♦ <u>The concerned tooth is absent;</u> ♦ Resembles OKC as keratin / parakeratin is formed <u>R/G</u> = R/L with a sclerotic borders in place of congenitally missing tooth; However, if formed from a supernumerary tooth bud, then no tooth is found absent from the arch, but it may give rise to lateral periodontal cyst appearance with some other tooth. <u>H/E</u> = basal cells are arranged as **picket-fence/ tombstone pattern,** i.e. same as OKC
Dentigerous/ follicular cyst (formation of **ameloblastoma** is far more common in DG cyst esp mural amelo. than in other odontogenic cysts)	Forms by fluid accumulation b/w REE and tooth crown; Involves crown of impacted/unerupted permanent tooth; Seldom a deciduous tooth is involved; Most common site is = third molars/max canines, as these are mostly impacted teeth. <u>Eruption cyst</u> = i.e. dilatation of normal follicular space about the crown of erupting tooth = is of deep blue color <u>Circumferential DG cyst</u> = i.e. surrounds the entire crown of tooth except occlusal surface <u>Paradental cyst</u> = arise i.r.t. to partly erupted vital tooth involved by pericoronitis;

Cysts (*Contd.*)

	H/E = p.o islands of odontogenic epith in the CT walls; can be mistaken for ameloblastoma; no rete pegs formed **Complications** = dev of **ameloblastoma**; epidermoid ca. and mucoepidermoid ca.
Apical PD/ radicular/PA cyst	Most common odontogenic cyst; due to caries & non-vital tooth; at the apex of the tooth; Residual cyst = a PA cyst left after the extraction. The epith lining is derived from epith rests of Malassez and so no amelo-blastoma-tous transformation.
Lateral PD cyst / an intraosseous lesion	Arises with the lateral root surface of the erupted tooth esp in mandibular premolar area; Originate as primordial cyst of supernumerary tooth, as there is high incidence of super-numerary tooth in this area; Gingival cyst of adults = also arises from post-functional dental lamina rests (extraosseous or peripheral lesion);
Botryoid odontogenic cyst	Multilocular; polycystic variant of lateral PD cyst. Associated Tooth is VITAL
Dental lamina cyst of newborn	Nodules on alveolar ridge of newborns; arise from remnants of dental lamina
Epstein's pearls	Found along midpalatal raphe; derived from entrapped epithelium along the line of fusion;
Bohn's nodules	At the junction of hard and soft palate; derived from palatal salivary gland structures; Are localised in the corium below the surface epithelium;
Gingival cyst of adults	2 types = 1. Arises from glands or rests of Serres (dental lamina) 2 arises from traumatic implantation.

Cysts (*Contd.*)

	3 arises from post-functional rests of dental lamina and so represents the extraosseous counterpart of lateral PD cyst. R/G = superficial erosion of cortical plate; a soft tissue lesion.
Odontogenic keratocyst OKC	♦ **Very high recurrence rate** ♦ Parakeratin = persisting nuclei; orthokeratin = no nuclei ♦ Str. granulosum is present in orthokeratin; not in parakeratin ♦ H/E = corrugated parakeratin surface;+ uniformly thick epithelium without rete pegs (6–10 cells thick) + **picket fence/ tombstone appearance** of basal layer; satellite / daughter cysts. Its epith is very active with marked growth potential/ mitotic activity ♦ C/F = 20–30 yrs age; in mand > maxillary; esp in ramal-3rd molar area; ass. with jaw cysts-basal cell nevus synd (multiple OKCs); lumen filled with thicker creamy mat/ keratin. ♦ Protein content of liquid is very low than serum. ♦ Rx = surgical excision, but very difficult due to friable lining and so recurrence. So a long term follow- up of 5 yrs is required.
Jaw cysts-basal cell nevus- bifid rib synd/Gorlin & Goltz synd	Hereditary, AD ♦ C/F = cutaneous anomalies = BCC, dermoid cysts/ tumors ♦ Dental/osseous anomalies = **multiple OKCs**; mild mand prognathism; bifid rib ♦ Ophthalmic = hypertelorism, etc. ♦ Neurologic = dural calcifications; ♦ Sexual = hypogonadism; ovarian tumors

Cysts (*Contd.*)

	♦ Lack of response to PTH and lack of PO 4 diuresis and 4th metacarpal shortening = related to pseudohypoparathyroidism ♦ Rx = high recurrence of OKCs, due to daughter/ satellite cysts found in the walls; ameloblastoma may develop
Calcifying odontogenic cyst/ Gorlin cyst	♦ It has features of both cyst and neoplasm ♦ 3 types = type 1A = simple unicystic type; intra / extra osseous/ focal areas of stellate reticulum present ♦ type 1B = odontome producing type; intra/ extraosseous; unilocular cyst; has formation of calcified material; ♦ type 1C = ameloblastomatous proliferating type; only intraosseous; ♦ type II = neoplasm like lesion; ameloblastoma like strands in CT wall; aka dentinoid-ghost cell tumor;

ECTODERMAL TUMORS

Enameloma/ enamel drop/ pearl	Arises due to misplaced ameloblasts; not a true neoplasm **Most common site** = bifurcation of the roots or near the CEJ
Ameloblastoma/ adamentinoma	True neoplasm which does not undergo differentiation to the point of enamel formation/no hard tissue is present in it. 1. Peripheral / extraosseous type = occurs in the soft tissues; 2. Pituitary / Rathke's pouch tumor = involves CNS; most common tumor of the childhood; destroys the pituitary; (Rathke's pouch arises from stomadeal ectoderm)

Ectodermal Tumors (*Contd.*)

	3. Malignant amelo- = i.e. metastatic; is well differentiated. 4. Ameloblastic ca. = malignant transformation of epithelial component; poorly differentiated C/F = mostly in mandible; in molar-ramal area; Expands the bone rather than perforating it; no breakdown of OMM; R/G = HONEY-COMB / SOAP-BUBBLE APPEARANCE; multilocular; thinning of cortices. H/E = 5 types- 1. Follicular/ simple = cystic degeneration of stellate reticulum. 2. Plexiform = cells arranged as irregular networks of interconnecting strands of cells 3. Acanthomatous = stellate reticulum undergoes squamous metaplasia 4. Granular = granules are lysosomal aggregates 5. Basal cell type = resembles BCC of skin; least common
Pindborg's tumor / CEOT	Is associated with impacted tooth; mainly in molar area of mandible R/G = **honeycomb pattern; driven-snow appearance** due to scattered flecks of calcification; H/E = origin = stratum intermedium; calcifications in the form of LIESEGANG RINGS;
Adenoamelo-blastoma/ adenomatoid odontogenic tumor	♦ Formation of duct like structures by epithelial components ♦ In U > L jaws; esp in anterior part of the jaws, due to accessibility of glands; anterior to max canines, ass. with impacted canines; ♦ R/G = unilocular R/L, resembling DG cyst but EXTENDS APICALLY FURTHER THAN THE CEJ.

MESODERMAL TUMORS

Peripheral odontogenic/ ossifying fibroma	Arises b/w teeth; has a calcified stalk; cuffing calcifications are found
Central odontogenic fibroma	More in children and young; H/E = fibro-blasts are very uniform in their placement & are usually **equidistant.**
Odontogenic myxoma	1. Arises from mesenchymal part of the tooth germ, i.e. dental papilla, follicle or PDL 2. Found only in jaws; not on other bones H/E = **mottled / honeycomb appearance** of bone; destructive Hyaluronic acid and chondroitin sulfate are found; Hyaluronic acid may be a significant factor in neoplastic behaviour; cells exhibit high alk Pase and LDH activity
Peripheral cemental dysplasia/ cementoma/ cementoblastoma	Lesion occurs in and near the PDL around apex of tooth, usually mand incisors, **involving multiple teeth**. Associated teeth are VITAL. R/G = 1. Osteolytic stage = periapical fibrosis, R/L same as PAP/ granuloma. 2. cementoblastic stage = calcific deposits start; increased cementoblastic activity 3. mature stage = R/O with a thin R/L line (same as condensing osteitis/ ch. focal sclerosing osteomylitis)
Central cementifying fibroma	L>U; displacement of teeth may be an early C/F. R/G = well circumscribed R/L or R/O or mixed; well demarcated from the surrounding bone; (as cp. to fibrous dysplasia which has diffuse R/G appearance)

Mesodermal Tumors (*Contd.*)

	♦ CCF and central ossifying fibroma and central cemento-ossifying fibroma = grow by expansion due to **centrifugal growth pattern** rather than a linear one. So it presents as a round tumor mass. When the mass reaches inferior mand border, the **expansion outline is in continuity** with outline of tumor mass above. Other lesions expand cortex linearly and outline of expanded mand is not in continuity with remainder of outline of lesion.
Benign cementoblastoma/ true cementoma	True neoplasm of cementoblasts, Ass. with VITAL TOOTH; R/G = mass is **attached to root**; is well circumscribes dense R/O surrounded by thin, uniform, R/L line; **Outine of affected root is obliterated** because of root resorption and fusion of the mass to the tissues.; **obliterated PDL.**
Dentinoma	Very rare; central in mandible; esp in molar area; ass. with an impacted tooth; H/E = **lack of enamel formation**; presence of irregular dentin ka osteodentin/ dentinoid. P.O. **undifferentiated odontogenic epith is characteristic**.

MIXED TUMORS OF ODONTOGENIC ORIGIN

Ameloblastic fibroma	No E and D formation; it does not form b/w trabeculae of bone, but it enlarges by gradual expansion so that periphery of lesion remains smooth.
Odontoma	Both ectodermal and mesenchymal cells exhibit complete differentiation, with abnor-

Mixed Tumors of Odontogenic Origin (*Contd.*)

	mal E and D formation; lack normal state of morpho-differentiation. ♦ **Compound** composite odontome = **resembles normal tooth** in anatomy; found in **anterior jaw**; ♦ **Complex** composite odontome = **irregular masses**; in **posterior jaw;** ♦ R/G = situated b/w the teeth; R/O with very thin R/L periphery
Ameloblastic odontoma	1. Simultaneously p.o. Ameloblastoma + composite odontoma; 2. A peculiar proliferation of tissues of odontogenic apparatus in unrestrained pattern, including complete morphodiff. + apposition + calcification. 3. R/G = p.o. many small R/O masses within the lesion which may / may not resemble teeth 4. H/E = unusual and characteristic; epith cells, ameloblasts, E/D/C, osteodentin, stellate reticulum like tissues, dental papilla, bone, ameloblastoma like H/E.
Teratoma	True neoplasm; made of tissues not native to that area in which the tumor occurs, e.g. ovary; non-odontogenic, but the teeth found in lesions which resemble the bicuspids.

<u>Periapical cemento-osseous dysplasia (PCOD) =</u>

- ♦ Ass. with VITAL teeth esp lower incisors;
- ♦ Predilection for females/ blacks
- ♦ R/G = 3 stages, i.e. osteolytic; cementoblastic and mature seen as R/L; mixed R/O; well circumscribed respectively.

<u>Focal COD (FCOD)</u> = most common fibro-osseous lesion;

- ♦ In Posterior mandible esp edentulous region;

- Well defined R/L or mixed or R/O
- Hemorrhagic; so **curettage is difficult;** (as cp to ossifying fibroma which is enucleated easily)

Florid COD = familial; in blacks;

- bilateral symmetrical involvement in posterior quadrant of the jaws;
- dull pain/ drainage, etc. are almost always ass. with exposure of sclerotic calcified masses to the oral cavity; causing chronic sclerosing osteomylitis and sequestrum formation
- R/G = sclerotic lobular masses symmetrically located in various areas of the jaws seen as CLOUD OF COTTON BALLS
- Prevent biopsy / extraction of the teeth

REGRESSIVE ALTERATIONS OF THE TEETH

Attrition	Physiologic wearing away of the tooth material; ass. with the aging process; first C/F = **polished facets,** decreases arch length as also occurs at proximal surfaces; Advanced attrition is seen in AI / DI.
Abrasion	Pathological wearing of tooth substances.; usually occurs at EXPOSED ROOT SURFACE OF THE TOOTH; as cementum is softer than enamel; Seen as a wedge-shaped ditch near CEJ; exposed dentin appears highly polished;
Erosion	Chemical loss of tooth material without involving bacterial action; Smooth, highly polished, scooped out depression on enamel adj to CEJ; Etio = citrate juices; gastric acidity; carbonated drinks; chronic vomiting esp in anorexia nervosa.

Regressive Alterations of the Teeth (*Contd.*)

Dental sclerosis/ transparent dentin	Calcification of dentinal tubules due to trauma, caries, etc. Decreased conductivity of odontoblastic processes. Shows an advancing carious process. Harder than adj. normal dentin
Dead tracts	Are not calcified and are permeable to penetration of dyes
Secondary dentin/irregular dentin	Aka adventitious dentin; deposited after the completion of primary dentin; ass. with normal aging process; aka **irritation dentin** as it is also stimulated by trauma, caries, attrition, etc. **Tertiary dentin** = localised exclusively adj to the irritated zone; tubules are less in number, v. irregular,
Pulp calcifications	1. **True denticles** = resemble dentin due to their tubular structure; resemble secondary dentin as tubules are less and irregular; more common in PULP CHAMBERS; 2. **Free denticles** = not attached to dentinal wall, but lying entirely in pulp tissues 3. **Attached denticles** = are continuous with dentinal wall; it is more common than free denticles; 4. **False denticles** = are localised masses of the calcified tissue and do not contain dentinal tubules. They are made of concentric layers of dentin. Are more common in pulp chamber and are larger than true denticles. 5. **Interstitial denticles** = when concentric apposition of calcified material continues and comes in apposition with dentinal wall. 6. **Diffuse calcifications** = most common in RCs; as calcific degenerates

Regressive Alterations of the Teeth (*Contd.*)

Resorption of teeth	**External R** = by PA granuloma; of reimplanted tooth (later on ankylosis occurs); by pressure of cysts (most common by apical PD cyst) and tumors; by heavy orthodontic forces; In **Hypothyroidism** = esp in patients receiving the orthodontic Rx. **Idiopathic R** = i.e. no known cause; mostly in maxillary premolars; central incisors; < 4 mm in size; **Internal R** = aka odontoclastoma; **pink tooth of Mummery**; Is due to inflammatory hyperplasia of the pulp;
Hypercementosis/ cementum hyperplasia	Deposition of Sec. Cementum/cellular, on the root surface; Increased in non-functional teeth; In **paget's disease** = generalised deposition of cementum occurs some distance away from the apex, because cementoblasts at apex have been lost by inflammatory process. **In paget's disease** = generalised deposition of sec. cementum at the roots occurs and APPARENT DISAPPEARANCE OF LAMINA DURA.
Cementicles	Foci of calcified tissue lie free in PDL; Dev. By calcification of nests of epith cell rests in PDL

DENTAL CARIES

1. Caries is a MULTIFACTORIAL DISEASE
2. Sucrose = most cariogenic
3. Urea = inhibitory substance to acid formation
4. Lactic acid is produced which = causes caries
5. Acidogenic theory is the most imp theory of caries

6. Sclerotic dentin is = caries resistant
7. Caries is the most prevalent disease of human race
8. Blacks have less caries than whites = due to dietary habits
9. Soft / processed food = increases caries
10. Caries in deciduous teeth = M > F
11. Caries in permanent teeth = F >M
12. It is due to difference in eruption times of the teeth and to the length of exposure of teeth to oral atmosphere
13. Water fluoridation = decreases caries

Etiology = 3 theories

1. Acidogenic theory (Miller's chemico-parasite theory)
2. Proteolytic theory
3. Proteolysis-chelation theory

Acidogenic theory

- Lactic acid is produced by = degradation of carbohydrates
- Strept mutans is the = main culprit; is ACIDURIC
- Actinomyces viscosus = root caries
- **First stage** = decalcification of **inorganic part** of E and D by lactic acid, resulting in its total destruction as a preliminary stage (chalky lesion is produced)
- **Second stage** = lysis of **organic part** by proteolytic enzymes
- Plaque (aka microcosm) is essential to hold = lactic acid on the tooth surface for initiation of caries.
- PH of plaque in caries free person = 7.3–7.6; and in caries active person = 4.5–5.5
- Acquired pellicle = forms from glycoproteins of saliva and serves as a nutrient for plaque microorganisms and help in plaque formation
- Plaque has much greater buffering capacity than saliva = due to p.o. HCO_3 ions and proteins.

- UREA = inhibits the decrease in plaque pH. It gets hydrolysed by bacterial enzyme, i.e. urease to ammonium carbonate, increases the neutralisation power of saliva and so a partial inhibition of pH drop is there.
- Time required for development of definite cavitation on enamel surface = approx 3 yrs.
- During **initiation of caries** = **Strept mutans** are more
- During **developing of the lesion** = **lactobacilli increase** in number.
- Sucrose in p.o. Strept mutans by **enz glucosyl transferase** gives → GLUCANS. They help in adherence of plaque to enamel and it is resistant to bacterial hydrolytic enz., acts as barrier vs the diffusion of salivary buffers and prevents neutralisation of acid formed in plaque.
- Saliva influences the acid production = less acid on mandibular Anterior teeth, so less caries (more calculus on maxillary molars and on mandibular Incisors).
- **Dextranase** produced by penicillium funiculosum = hydrolysis dextrans/glucans and minimizes plaque formation and prevents smooth surface caries.

Anticaries agents

1. Urea
2. Dextranase from penicillium funiculosum
3. Ammonia
4. Fluorides
5. Thiocyanate ions were thought to help inhibit the bacteria associated with caries.
6. Vit. B deficiency = may exert **caries-protective effect** on the tooth.
7. Vit. B_6 / pyridoxine = is anticaries; it selectively alters the oral flora
8. PO_4^- are effective cariostatic agents
9. Increase in Vanadium, V = decrease caries

Proteolytic theory; by Gottlieb

- Here, **organic part** is attacked first, i.e. proteolysis (more in rod sheath than lamellae)
- Then, acid enters the roughened enamel rods for **decalcification of the inorganic part**.
- Enamel lamellae and E. rods sheath have organic part = serve as pathway for microbes
- Enamel has 0.56 % organic part; esp **KERATIN** (dentin has COLLAGEN)
- **Yellow pigmentation** of caries is due to = pigments produced by proteolytic bacteria.
- EARLY CARIES LESION = microscopic phase of caries, i.e. bacteria beneath an apparently **intact enamel surface** and extend laterally in enamel.
- **$CaSO_4$ is found in carious enamel** and not in sound enamel. It is produced by enz sulfanase from some G (-) bact; breaks enamel mucoproteins to form H_2SO_4.

Proteolytic-chelation theory: by Schatz

- Chelation = formation of complexes with metallic ions, e.g. chlorophyll, Hb, tetracycline, etc.
- Most common biologic chelating agent = citrate

Mechanism of action =

- Both inorganic and organic parts of the tooth are attacked simultaneously.
- Keratinolytic bacteria attack organic part esp keratin of enamel. Substances thus formed form chelates with inorganic components of tooth and cause decalcification.
- **Lactobacillus count** increases = this bact is the **result of caries**, rather than the cause.
- Proteolysis provides ammonia, which prevents drop in pH, and tends to inhibit the growth of lactobacilli.
- Release of Ca^{2+} from HA = encourages the growth of lactobacilli.

- Fluorides = form fluorapatite with HA, which strengthens the enamel.
- Incorporation of **chelating agents, e.g. EDTA**, in cariogenic diet results in **increase in severity of caries**.

Prominent points

- Surface enamel is more resistant to caries than sub surface enamel.
- Surface enamel is more highly mineralised and has F, Zn, Pb, Fe, lower in CO_2, dissolves at slower rate in acids, has more organic material and less water = slow disintegration.
- Deep P and F on surfaces = more caries.
- With attrition, flat surface = less caries.
- Conc. of Ca and P is more in slow-flowing saliva; and is low in caries-active patient.
- Greater ammonia content of saliva of caries immune patients = retard plaque formation and neutralise acids.

Saliva

- most prominent and important oral enzyme = amylase / ptyaline, which degrades starch.
- **Parotid saliva has a higher conc**. of amylase content than saliva from other glands
- Xerostomia / salivary gland aplasia => rampant caries
- **Resting saliva** = i.e. the amount of saliva constantly being secreted by salivary glands
- Viscosity = high caries in thick, mucinous saliva
- Viscosity of saliva = is due to high mucin content derived from submand, subling and accessory glands.
- Saliva contains antibacterial substance, i.e. lysozyme.
- Bacteriolytic factor in saliva which is ass. with globulin fraction of saliva = is active vs strept. and lactobacilli;
- Buffer capacity of saliva = acid neutralising power
- CO_2 capacity of caries-free saliva is more.

- Plaque acts as a barrier to buffer ions of saliva to reach the acid on tooth surface.
- Soft diet, more sticky, less mastication, less roughness, less attrition = > more caries.
- Mastication of food = decreases the number of oral bacteria.
- Not all sugars have same cariogenicity.
- Vit. A deficiency = affects developing teeth
- Vit. D deficiency = enamel hypoplasia
- Rickets = alteration in tooth structure, which increases the caries.
- Vit. K = tested for a possible anticaries agent by virtue of its enzyme-inhibiting activity in carbohydrate degradation cycle.
- Vit. B complex = malnourished patient has lower caries increment than well-nourished patient.
- Vit. B deficiency = may exert caries-protective effect on the tooth because vit. B is essential for growth for oral bacteria and serve as components of coenzymes involved in glycolysis.
- Vit. B_6 / pyridoxine = is anticaries; it selectively alters the oral flora by promoting growth of non-cariogenic bacteria which suppress the cariogenic forms.
- Vit. C deficiency = damage to pulps and PD tissues. No association with caries
- Ca and P metabolic disturbances during tooth formation → severe enamel hypoplasia and defects of dentition
- PO_4^- are effective cariostatic agents when added to diets cariogenic for lab rodents and depends on anions and cations with which they are combined. The mechanism operates after the teeth have erupted.
- Some evidence that Ca and P retention may be related to inactivity/ arrest of caries.
- Fluorides
- Increase in Selenium, Se = increases caries
- Increase in Vanadium, V = decrease caries
- Caries in blacks < whites; due to dietary habits

- Environmental factors have greater influence on caries than genetic factors
- Genetic = twins have resemblance; inheritance of tooth form or structure
- Pregnancy = fetal teeth do not calcify at the expense of mother's teeth.

CLINICAL ASPECTS OF DENTAL CARIES

1. **Primary / virgin caries**
2. **Secondary / recurrent caries**
3. **Pits and fissures caries** development does not depend on development of plaque; but smooth surface caries is preceded by plaque.
4. **Proximal caries** begins just below contact points, as faint, white opacity of enamel without loss of continuity; early white chalky spots become slightly **rough** due to superficial decalcification of enamel. It appears BLUISH-WHITE, when caries penetrates enamel esp when spreads along DEJ.
5. Spread of caries in P& F is rapid; but on smooth surface is SLOW.
6. **Cervical caries** from area opposite the gingival crest to convexity of tooth surface (i.e. up to self-cleansing area); is **crescent-shaped,** is always an open cavity; is directly / totally due to LACK OF ORAL HYGIENE.
7. **Recurrent caries** occurs immediately near to the restorations; due to leaky margins; improper removal of caries. In sealed dentinal tubules, lactobacilli die out but streptococci persist which cause caries.
8. **Arrested caries** occurs only on occlusal surfaces; is an open cavity the dentin gets burnished giving brown stained polished appearance and hard which is ka EBURNATION OF DENTIN; lesion becomes static; dentinal sclerosis occurs; also caries gets arrested by FLUORIDES.
9. **Incipient caries** lesion is smooth chalky white area as an area of decalcification beneath the dental plaque.

10. Differences-

Acute dental caries	**Chronic dental caries**	**Nursing bottle caries**
Rapid spread	**Slow**, involves pulp late	Aka **baby bottle syndrome** or bottle mouth synd
Mostly in **children** and young adults because dentinal tubules are large and open;	Mostly in **adults**; dentinal sclerosis	Affects **deciduous teeth** esp max incisors > max first molars > max canines;
Large internal cavitation	No undermining of enamel	
Pin point exposure	**Large entrance**	
No secondary dentin	May be there	
Dentin is stained light-yellow;	Deep brown color; minimum softening of dentin	**no caries in mand incisors** as they are covered by tongue and saliva, (as cp to rampant caries)
Pain present	Painless	

11. Pits and fissures are very prone to caries = because of very thin enamel at the base.
12. Enamel may appear opaque bluish white = due to undermining which occurs through lateral spread at DEJ.
13. Progress of a lesion which is open and exposed to oral cavity to saliva = is slower and pulp involvement is delayed.

Early enamel remineralisation

Caries reversibility can be achieved but: it occurs only when **cavitation does not occur.**

1. $CaPO_4$ solutions = causes hardening of surface
2. 1 ppm Fluoride solution = accelerates rate of deposition of $CaPO_4$ and hardening by forming FLUORAPATITE.

Caries susceptibility:

- U > L teeth, because saliva buffers the L teeth
- R and L are equal; bilateral.
- First molars are = most susceptible
- L incisors and canines = least susceptible
- Occlusal surface > M > D > B > L surfaces in susceptibility
- B > L caries in mandibular molars and L > B caries in maxillary molars; due to p.o. grooves and pits.

Histopathology of caries

A. Surface caries/Caries of enamel = earliest manifestation is incipient caries.

First change = loss of interprismatic or inter-rod substances of enamel

Increase prominence of rods and roughening of enamel rod ends.

So prisms are more susceptible to early attacks.

Transverse striations of enamel rods appear.

Accentuation of incremental striae of Retzius = due to loss of minerals and prominence of organic structure is the earliest change.

Shape = TRIANGULAR

Apex at DEJ; base at surface of the tooth

Surface of the enamel is rough.

4 zones = from dentin outwards are : **TDBS**

Zone I	Zone II	Zone III	Zone IV
Transluscent zone	Dark zone; aka positive zone	Body of lesion	Surface zone
Advancing front of the lesion	Forms due to deminer-alisation	Greatest deminer-alisation	Unaffected relatively
Slightly more porous than enamel			More resistant due to more mineralisation
Pore volume =1 %	2–4 %	5–25 %	5 %
% age demineralis-ation = 1–2 %	5–6 %	20–25 %	1–10 %
R/G = R/O	R/L	R/L	R/O

B. Pits and fissure caries

- Shape = triangular or cone shape = apex at outer surface; base at DEJ, i.e. along the directions of enamel rods.
- More number of dentinal tubules are involved at DEJ
- Greater cavitation than proximal smooth surface caries.
- More undermining of enamel.

CARIES OF DENTIN

Spreads along the DEJ; dentinal tubules act as tracts to pulp.

Five Zones of carious dentin = from pulp outwards to dentin, i.e. FSDID

I = fatty degeneration of Tome's fibres (is the first change)

II = dentinal sclerosis

III = decalcification of dentin

IV = bacterial invasion; intact but decalcified dentin.

V = decomposed dentin

It shows the progression towards the pulp, i.e. caries is advanced at DEJ and progressing towards the pulp. The first change seen is the fatty degeneration of Tome's granular layer.

Changes in the dentin

- dentinal sclerosis / transparent dentin forms, i.e. calcification of dentinal tubules which seals them *vs.* further penetration.
- fatty degeneration of Tome's dentinal fibres-fat contributes to impermeability of the dentinal tubules
- caries destruction rate is slower in adults due to sclerosis
- decalcification of dentin is slightly in advance to bacterial invasion.
- <u>Pioneer bacteria,</u> i.e. bacteria in dentinal tubules before any clinical evidence of carious process
- <u>Initial decalcification</u> involves walls of tubules; which get distended and filled with bacteria of one species/pure form, e.g. cocci or bacilli, etc.
- **Proteolytic bacteria predominate in deeper dentin caries**
- **Acidogenic bacteria predominate in early caries.**
- **Bacteria if sealed in tubules = strept persist; lactobacilli die**
- So initiation and progression of caries are DISTINCT PROCESSES.

In **dentinal tubules** = the changes seen are

- Thickening and swelling of the sheath of Neumann occurs.
- Increased diameter of tubule due to packing of bacteria
- Confluence of tubules occurs
- Liquefaction foci appear = are parallel to the dentinal tubules
- P. O. of globular dentin – helps on rapid caries spread in **malachotic teeth / soft teeth.**
- Decalcification by acidogenic bacteria

- Matrix destruction by proteolytic enzymes which has maximum activity only when organic matrix is decalcified; has **very little effect on intact dentin.**
- **Clefts / focal areas** appear in dentin perpendicular to the tubules, are parallel to contour lines of dentin.
- Clefts account for the peeling away of dentin by **excavation**
- Secondary dentin involvement = is very slow because of decreased number of tubules / irregular course.
- Spread of caries at the junction of primary and sec. dentin = LATERAL

ROOT CARIES: aka ***caries of cementum***

- Exposure of root surface is a must for initiation, that is why it is found mostly in later age group, when root gets exposed.
- Bacteria involved are = filamentous; **actinomyces viscosus**
- Bacteria invade along the Sharpey's fibres; spread laterally b/w various layers because cementum is lamellated structure.
- Decalcification is followed by matrix degeneration.
- Rate of caries progress is slower in root dentin due to less number of tubules
- **Most affected teeth** = mand first molars > mand premolars > max canines
- **Least affected teeth** = mand incisors
- I / D surfaces affected most frequently in U teeth
- Buccal surfaces affected most frequently in L teeth.

Methods of caries control

a. chemical measures

1. Substances which alter the tooth surface or structure, e.g. fluorides, chlorhexidine, alexidine, bisguanides, silver nitrate, zinc chloride, k-ferrocyanide, etc.
2. Substances which interfere with carbohydrate degradation, e.g. vit K, sarcosides

3. Substances which interfere with bacterial growth and metabolism, e.g. urea, ammonium compounds, combination of 5% amm. Compounds and 3 % urea is more effective.

FLUORIDES

- DEAN et al 1941, studied in Bauxite, Arkansas.
- 1 ppm fluoride should be used
- **Grands Rapids** = first city of water fluoridation 1945, January
- **first artificial fluoridation** = Newberg , New York, 1945 May
- DMF rate decreased by 60 %

Mechanism of action of fluorides : by 3 means, i.e.

1. F **inhibits the enzyme ENOLASE** and inhibits conversion of 2-PGA to phosphopyruvic acid; so prevents carbohydrate degradation.
2. F does not act by inhibitor of microbes, i.e. *Lactobacillus acidophillus*.
3. During the tooth formation, F combines with HA to form FA, i.e. fluorapatite, which is acid resistant.
4. Topical F = enamel adsorbs F on its surface through formation of CaF_2 / Ca-fluorapatite. For it , 8 % SnF_2 is the best, also 2% NaF and 1.23% APF is also used.

KNUTSON TECHNIQUE

- **2 % NaF is applied at** the age of 3,7,11, and 13 years of age, i.e. 4 applications every 3 years, i.e. total of 12 applications, because teeth erupt at this age phases. 40–45 % reduction in caries ;
- 8 % SnF_2 = single yearly application is used; is a very good technique;
- 1.23 % APF gel aka BRUDEVOLD'S SOLUTION, helps in greater F uptake by enamel.
- SnF_2 – PO_4 combination is better than SnF_2 and APF alone.
- SnF_2 in prophylaxis paste = 30–40 % decrease in caries.
- Most effective mass reduction of caries = by communal F action

F mouthwashes = 2 techniques, i.e.

1. High frequency–low potency technique = for home use
2. Low frequency–high potency technique = for school-based programmes

BISGUANIDES and alexidine, e.g.

chlorhexidine 0.2 % = is anticaries, antiplaque

- Gets adsorbed on tooth surface and salivary mucins and then it is released very slowly in an active form.
- But causes the discoloration of teeth.

SILVER NITRATE = Ag plugs the enamel lamellae and / or combines with soluble pathways of enamel to form a less soluble combination.

ZINC CHLORIDE and POT. FERRICYANIDE = gets impregnated in the enamel and seal off invasion pathways – but it is little clinical value.

SUBSTANCES WHICH INTERFERE WITH CARBOHYDRATE DEGRADATION:

1. Synthetic vit K = prevents acid formation
2. Sarcosides = are enzyme inhibitors / anti-enzymes; penetrate the plaque and prevent decrease in pH < 5.5, e.g. sodium N-lauryl sarcosinate, sod dehydroacetate. Palmityl compounds are better than lauroyl.

SUBSTANCES WHICH INTERFERE WITH BACTERIAL GROWTH and METABOLISM

1. **Urea and ammonium compounds** = prevent acid formation; decrease oral bacteria; bacteriostatic; salivary pH increases to > 8 after urea-quinine rinse. Urea releases ammonia gas by enz urease, which neutralises acids and interfere with bacterial growth.

NUTRITIONAL MEASURES

- Restrict carbohydrates, soft sticky foods, decrease the frequency of eating;

- Phosphated diet, e.g. 2 % dibasic Ca-PO_4; 1% sod. dihydrogen PO_4;
- Sod. DHP is better than $CaPO_4$ due to greater systemic action of sodium salts.
- Ca-sucrose PO_4 = penetrates the surface crystalline layers of enamel, tightening the attachments b/w crystals and protection of enamel vs acid disintegration.

MECHANICAL MEASURES

- BRUSHING = acid production in plaque occurs within minutes after ingestion of carbohydrates.
- Mouth rinsing = 0.2 % chlorhexidine; it is antibacterial and antiplaque
- Fluoride mouthwashes
- Flosssing = for cleaning proximal surfaces
- Detergent foods = fibrous foods; help in mechanical cleansing of teeth.
- P and F sealants, e.g. BIS-GMA, cyanoacrylates, etc.
- **Prophylactic odontotomy** = to make P and F self-cleansing

DISEASES OF PULP AND PA TISSUES

Anachoretic pulp = bacterial infection of intact pulp through vascular channels.

Aerodontalgia = pain at high altitude associated with esp recently filled teeth.

Focal reversible pulpitis/pulp hyperemia	Mild, transient, localised to the pulpal ends of irritated dentinal tubules; sensitive to COLD, pain disappears on removal of stimulus;
Acute pulpitis & acute	Severe pain by thermal changes esp by cold/ ice. Pain persists after removal of stimulus

Diseases of Pulp and Pa Tissues

Exacerbation of chronic pulpitis	**Pain increases when patient lies down.** Intrapulpal abscess formation → severe lancinating pain. Small opening of the lesion → no escape of inflammatory exudate so pressure leads to LIQUEFACTION necrosis and abscess; aka acute suppurative pulpitis.
Chronic pulpitis	Painless; necrotic pulp; wide opening to the lesion; **No thermal sensitivity** Ulcerative pulpitis = attempt by pulp to wall off the infection by forming collagen around inflammed area. It may resemble formation granulation tissue.
Chronic hyperplastic pulpitis/pulp polyp	Esp in children and young adults with large open carious lesion; Teeth esp D, E, 6 are involved; Insensitive to manipulation due to few nerves.
Gangrenous necrosis of pulp	Tissue destruction due to ischemia with superimposed bacterial infection by SAPROPHYTIC ORGANISMS.
PA granuloma; apical periodontitis	Tender to percussion due to inflammation of apical PDLR/G = earliest change is THICKENING OF PDL at apex. Outline of the R/L is diffuse in the bone = acute condition H/E = mainly macrophages, lymphocytes, plasma cells, i.e. an IMMUNE-TYPE GRANULOMA. Ig +ve, B-lymphocytes and plasma cells, mainly IgG. Russell **bodies** may be present. Non-B lymphocytes are probably T-cells = so lesion could be a delayed type of hypersensitivity reaction.

Diseases of Pulp and Pa Tissues (*Contd.*)

	FOAM CELLS = large number of phagocytes ingest lipid material. **Cholesterol crystals** = seen as clear needle-like spaces or clefts (which are common in lesions with MNGCs and cyst formation). Main bacteria = *S. viridans, Str. hemolyticus, Staph. aureus*.
Apical PD cyst / radicular cyst/ PA cyst / root end cyst	True cyst as it is lined by epithelium derived from rests of Malassez. Cells proliferate at the periphery and cells in the central part get separated from the nutrition, degenerate and liquefy; Epith lining is stratified squamous. **Rushton body** or hyaline body = found in greater number in epith of PA cysts → arise from thrombus formation by RBCs, i.e. a **rouleux phenomenon.** Universal occurrence of inflammatory infiltérate in CT = made of lymphocytes and plasma cells + PMN cells Diff. b/w PA cyst and PA granuloma = P.O. epith-lined lumen in the cyst.
Residual cyst	May develop if epith remnants remain after enucleation of cyst

OSTEOMYELITIS

Acute suppurative osteo.	Diffuse spread of infection throughout the medullary spaces, with subsequent necrosis of bone. **Most common bacteria** = *Staph. aureus; Staph. albus* R/G = individual trabeculae become *fuzzy*, indistinct, and R/L areas develop.

Osteomyelitis (*Contd.*)

	Trabeculae may loose their viability and undergo slow resorption. **Sequestrum** = i.e. bone which has lost its vitality begins to separate from living bone is ka sequestrum. **Involucrum** = i.e. when sequestrum gets surrounded by new living bone.
Chronic focal sclerosing osteo./ condensing osteitis	Reactionary bone formation in case of chronic infections or very high tissue resistance. Almost occurs in young age, i.e. < 20 yrs, esp in mand 1st molar area. Occurs as a reaction of bone to mild bacterial reaction in patients with high tissue resistance. R/G = well circumscribed R/O mass of sclerotic bone surrounding root apex; this **sclerotic bone is not attached to tooth** and remains in bone after the tooth is removed-it is ka <u>bone scar/residual</u> CFSO. Also, entire root outline is always visible (as cp to benign cementoblastoma)
Chronic diffuse sclerosing osteo. CDSO	Proliferation reaction of bone to low grade infections; Portal of entry = through diffuse PD disease Most common in older, edentulous, mandibular, blacks, female patients, R/G = resembles paget's dis = **cotton wool appearance**, borders b/w lesions and normal bone are INDISTINCT. H/E = dense, irregular trabeculae lined by osteoblasts; sclerotic avascular bone; **mosaic pattern** of bone; Rx = lesion is too extensive to be removed surgically;

Osteomyelitis (*Contd.*)

	Rx of choice = If a tooth is present in the sclerotic bone, then extraction + liberal amount of bone should be removed to **induce fresh bleeding**.
Sclerotic cemental masses (SCM)	Multiple symmetrical lesions; resembling CDSO H/E = tissue is cementum, smooth, with globular accretion pattern; sclerotic cementum
Florid osseous dysplasia	Simultaneous occurrence of multiple SIMPLE BONE CYSTS; along with CDSO and SCM type lesions. It is due to abnormal reaction of bone to irritation
Chronic osteo. With proliferating periosteitis/ Garre's chronic non – suppurative sclerosing osteitis/ periosteitis ossificans	It is **focal thickening** of bone due to peripheral reactive bone formation due to chronic soft tissue infection/cellulitis. Mostly on anterior surface of tibia and on outer surface of cortex of mandible ka DUPLICATION OF CORTICAL LAYER OF BONE. The mass is smooth, well calcified and shows a thin but definite cortical layer, H/E = SUPRACORTICAL but subperiosteal; Trabeculae are perpendicular to cortex; but parallel to each other. D/D = Caffey's disease, hypervitaminosis A, syphilis, leukemia, Ewing's sarcoma, metastatic neuroblastoma, fracture callus.

RADIOGRAPHIC FEATURES OF DIFFERENT OSTEOMYELITIS

Acute suppurative osteomyelitis	♦ Initiallly = no change ♦ After 2–3 wks = diffuse lytic changes in bone

Radiographic features of different osteomyelitis (*Contd.*)

	♦ Individual trabeculae appear = fuzzy and indistinct ♦ R/L areas start developing = Moth-eaten appearance / subperiosteal deposition (granular densification) ♦ Sequestrum appear = if bone is formed around it, it is ka involucrum ♦ Sequestrum is more R/O than living bone = because of metastatic calcifications and due to demineralisation type appearance when new blood vessels appear.
Chronic suppurative osteomyelitis	♦ Somewhat same as above, but fistulae and sinus develop
Chronic focal sclerosing osteo/ condensing osteitis	♦ Well circumscribed, DISTINCT from adj.... Bone, R/O masses of sclerotic bone; around & extending down from the root of the involved carious tooth. ♦ Entire **root outline is visible** (as cp to benign cementoblastoma) ♦ Sclerotic bone not attached to tooth, remains in bone after the tooth is removed – it is ka **bone scar** / residual CFSO.
Chronic diffuse sclerosing osteo	♦ Diffuse sclerosis R/O areas in bone; ♦ Border b/w sclerosis and normal bone is INDISTINCT. ♦ May mimic **Paget's disease = cotton wool appearance**
Chronic osteomyelitis with proliferative periosteitis	♦ Focal overgrowth of bone on outer surface of cortex, described as duplication of cortical layer of bone; ♦ Mass is smooth, well calcified, with **a thin but definite cortical layer**; may show **onion peel appearance.**

SPREAD OF ORAL INFECTIONS

Cellulitis = mainly caused by streptococci; inflammation spreads along the fascial planes; the organisms produce FIBROLYSINS AND HYALURONIDASES;

The maxillary infections = perforate outer cortex ABOVE THE BUCCINATOR and cause swelling of upper half of face initially.

The mandibular infections = perforate BELOW THE BUCCINATOR and cause swelling of lower half of face.

1. INFRATEMPORAL SPACE

Inferior part of ITS is ka PTERYGOMANDIBULAR SPACE. It lies b/w mesial pterygoid m and ramus. Its infection is due to pericoronitis of mand 3rd molars.

2. POST–ZYGOMATIC SPACE = extends antero-medially from ITS.

Contents = pterygoid plexus; internal maxillary A; external pterygoid m.; mandibular N; nerves to mylohyoid, buccinator ms; and lingual N, chorda tympani N.

Swelling of eyelid occurs esp if post-zygomatic fossa is involved.

3. Space of body of the mandible = is enclosed by a layer of fascia derived from deep cervical fascia which splits at its lower border.

Infections of I, C, PM = cause induration of labial sulcus if outer cortical plate is involved. and of floor of mouth if inner cortical plate is involved.

In case of infections of molars

- Involves outer cortex = if infection perforates above the external oblique line (EOL), i.e. the buccinator attachment.
- Skin perforation = if perforates below the EOL
- Floor of mouth = if above the mylohyoid attachment
- Submaxillary space or lateral pharyngeal space = if below the mylohyoid attachment.

4. Submasseteric space = lies b/w masseter and ramus. It is parallel to middle part of the muscle and extends U and B b/w middle and deep part. It gets involved by mand 3rd molar infection via retromolar fossa.

5. SUBMANDIBULAR SPACE = has 3 spaces, i.e. submaxillary and sublingual and submental spaces. The infection may spread contralaterally by extension anterior to the HYOGLOSSUS ms.

(a) Submaxillary space = lies medial to mandible and below POST PART OF MYLOHYOID m; gets infected by mand molars infection; is one of the most commonly involved.

(b) Sublingual space = lies below mucosa of floor of mouth and ABOVE THE MYLOHYOID; situated above the submaxillary space; gets involved by infection perforating the lingual cortical plate above the mylohyoid attachment.

(c) Submental space = limited in depth by mylohyoid;

6. LUDWIG'S ANGINA = esp by STREPTOCOCCI

Bilateral involvement of all the submandibular spaces; cellulitis begins mainly in submaxillary space due to 2nd and 3rd molars as their APICES ARE SITUATED BELOW THE MYLOHYOID RIDGE.

Infection of sublingual space is common by 1st molars = as its apices are ABOVE THE MYLOHYOID RIDGE.

C/F = board like swelling of floor of mouth; deviation of tongue,

7. CAVERNOUS SINUS THROMBOSIS =

Infection of face is carried by facial and angular Vs;

Infection spreading through external route is RAPID = due to large open system of Vs leading directly to the sinus.

Infection spreading through internal / pterygoid route is slow.

Focal infections

Rh fever = develops due to an altered reactivity or hypersensitivity of tissues to hemolytic streptococci.

High conc of Abs to Ag of the hemolytic streptococci group are found in these patients.

One of the most striking feature of cultures from teeth during RCT is = relative infrequency of occurrence of hemolytic streptococci.

Hemolytic streptococci are = most imp in causing Rh arthritis and Rh fever.

The patient has high Ab titre to hemolytic streptococci = suggest the hypersensitivity reaction.

Bacteremia = esp caused by *Strept. viridans*.

Microbes most commonly involved in UTI = *E. coli; Strept. hemolyticus*.

PHYSICAL AND CHEMICAL INJURIES

Ultraspeed is best; water cooling is must; low pressure must be applied;

Speeds of > 50,000 rpm with coolants are less injurious to the pulp than lower speeds;

ZOE is least injurious of all the filling materials.

Resins = injurious agent is residual MONOMER; marginal leakage is due to shrinkage; heat is generated during the setting.

Polycarboxylate and polyacrylate cements are less irritant to the pulp;

GI cements are polyacrylate based – are biocompatible and anticaries.

If more than 2 mm of primary dentin remains b/w restoration and pulp, then dentin itself provides insulation.

If less than 2 mm — then cement base should be used.

Cavity liners = are aqueous or volatile organic liquid suspensions of ZnO or $Ca(OH)_2$ or solutions of resins in an organic solvent to which ZnO or $Ca(OH)_2$ have been added. They neutralize the free acids of $ZnPO_4$ and silicate cements.

Cavity varnishes = decrease post-operative sensitivity; are solutions of one or more resins from natural gums, synthetic resins or rosin in organic solvents. Its film does not provide thermal insulations but acts as a semipermeable membrane. Decreases the microleakage.

Cavity primers = increase the adaptation of MMA filling materials to cavity walls and help in providing marginal seal.

BRUXISM = night grinding

Bruxomania = day grinding

In children; this habit is frequently associated with the transition from deciduous to the permanent dentition.

FRACTURES OF TEETH = esp in children with C2 D1 m.o.; males; maxillary teeth

Ellis's classification =

Class I = only enamel

Class II = enamel and dentin

Class III = enamel, dentin and pulp

Class IV = non-vital with / without loss of crown structure

Class V = tooth loss

Class VI = fracture of root with / without loss of crown structure

Class VII = displacement of tooth

Class VIII = fracture of crown en –masse and its replacement

Class IX = trauma to a deciduous tooth.

Root fractures are uncommon in young children = because their roots are incompletely formed and teeth have some resilience in the sockets.

Fracture of tooth is less damaging than non-fracture = as whole force of trauma is not dissipated to the investing tissues.

Healing = most satisfactory healing occurs by **calcific union**.

If the apposition b/w the 2 segments is not close = then healing is by CT / fibrous alone. The cells come from pulp and PDL.

Ankylosis = of deciduous teeth is ka SUBMERGED TOOTH.

It is the fusion of root to the bone through the cementum or bone, during healing of root resorption. Mainly occurs due to trauma. On percussion, a dull, muffled sound is heard. On R/G., loss of PDL space in the area of ankylosis.

Traumatic cyst (solitary bone / haemorrhagic / unicameral / extravasation / simple bone cyst)

- Not lined by epithelium
- Due to trauma to bone, so intermedullary hemorrhage occurs, clot does not reorganize. Degeneration of clot leads to cavity formation.

- It contains only air but not blood (only lesions which contain blood are aneurysmal bone cyst, hemangioma and sometimes central giant cell granulomas).
- Size of cavity increases by edema due to restriction of venous drainage.
- Associated teeth are VITAL.
- Occurs esp in mand. posterior area.
- Intracystic hydrostatic pressure is very low.
- R/G = lamina dura of teeth is INTACT = vital teeth
- It **lies above the mandibular canal**; but lingual salivary gland depression (Stafne's cyst) lies below the mandibular canal.
- **Rx = re-establish the bleeding in the space lesion.**
- **Lamina dura** is a thin white R/O shadow outlining the tooth sockets. It is the thin layer of dense bone the so called cribriform plate or alveolar bone proper. This bone is a layer cortical bone / bundle bone; is little thicker — with no more highly mineralised than trabeculae of cancellous bone.

Effects of OTM

- New trabeculae on the tension side have thin, elongated spicules arranged parallel to PDL fibres;
- Bone gets resorbed than cementum = because bone is vascular but cementum is avascular;
- OTM in younger is more rapid than in older patients = because in old / increasing age the vascularity of bone decreases.
- In intrusive movement = new bone formation is actually minimal
- With movement of deciduous teeth = permanent teeth moves in that direction; so shape of permanent dental arch can be modified by altering the deciduous arch.

PHYSICAL INJURIES OF SOFT TISSUES

- Traumatic ulcers = aka decubitus ulcers
- Factitial injuries = are accidentally self induced injuries due to some habits

- Traumatic ulcer = aka sore spots
- **Denture stomatitis** = aka denture sore mouth; is not a true allergy but due to *Candida albicans*; redness is restricted to the area in contact with denture
- **Inflammatory fibrous hyperplasia / epulis fissuratum** = i.e. hyperplasia along the borders of dentures; is due to chronic irritation of denture flanges; PLASMA pooling, i.e. muco-polysaccharides keratin dystrophy of surface epithelium in the spinous layer is seen.
- Inflammatory papillary hyperplasia / **palatal papillomatosis** = seen in palatal mucosa as red inflammatory papillary projections; H/E = vertical projections with CT cores; chronic sialoadenitis of accessory glands.
- **Perleche** / angular cheilitis / angular cheilosis = by *Candida albicans*; due to overclosure of jaws and saliva collects in the folds at corners of mouth; also by riboflavin deficiency. The deep fissures and cracks stop at the MUCOCUTANEOUS JUNCTIONS.
- **Mucocele** = is due to severance of the duct of the <u>minor salivary glands</u>. Most frequently on lower lip; extravasation type is more common than the retention mucocele / true cyst. **Mucocele is restricted almost to lower lip** and seldom on upper lip; while accessory SG neoplasms of lips are almost universally present on the upper lips.
- True retention mucocele is lined by epithelium, the epithelial lining is the epith of the FEEDER DUCT of the injured SG. Rx = excision with removal of the associated SG.
- **Ranula** = occurs in floor of mouth ass with ducts of submand / sublingual glands; is painless; on one side of the floor of mouth; mucosa appears as bluish color;
- **Sialolithiasis** = i.e. salivary duct stone; are due to deposition of calcium salts esp $CaPO_4$; C/F = pain is due to collection of saliva during meals and swelling of glands. It is **most common in submand SG** (64%), which is due to tenacity of its saliva with high MUCIN contents and long irregular course of the duct.

CHEMICAL INJURIES

• Drug allergy = ka stomatitis medicamentosa

• Contact stomatitis = is stomatitis venenata

• $AgNO_3$ = is used as **caries preventing**; chemical cautery and sterilising solution.

• **Bismuth line** = a thin blue black line in marginal gingiva; which is sometimes confined to gingival papillae. Pigment is bismuth sulfide precipitates in the tissues where H_2S gas is formed esp in the areas of food stagnation. It Rx is = contramine and BAL.

• **Phenytoin** = causes fibrous hyperplasia (also by nifedipin; cyclosporin); stimulates wound healing due to proliferation of fibroblasts and increased collagen synthesis. H/E = rete pegs are extremely long and thin and aka TEST TUBE PEGS.

• **Lead poisoning** = aka **plumbism**; a **peripheral neuritis** may develop which produce the characteristic WRIST-DROP / FOOT-DROP.

Blood changes are = hypochromic anemia; with BASOPHILIC STIPPLING OF RBCs.

• **Lead line** = aka **Burtonian line**; is gray/bluish line roound the gingival margin. H_2O_2 turns it in white line.

Lead may get deposited in deciduous teeth, which serve as an index of body burden of lead.

Rx = sodium calcium edetate.

• **Mercury** = patient has fine tremors of fingers; limbs; lips and tongue, remarkably increased saliva flow, i.e. **ptyalism.**

Rx = dimercaprol; BAL

• **Acrodynia** = aka **Pink's disease** / Swift's disease

Is due to mercurial toxicity; most common in young infants of < 2 yrs age; skin resembles RAW- BEEF; skin peeling; severe pruritis; **children tear their hair out in patches**. Rx = BAL, i.e. British anti-lewisite

• Silver = **argyria**; argyrosis. Ag granules are prominently arranged in linear fashion along the collagen fibres and around blood vessels, etc.

TETRACYCLINE STAINING = avoid during first 7–8 yrs of life as teeth are developing during that time.

- It is due to complex / chelate formation with calcium in teeth/ bone.
- It crosses the placental barrier.
- On deciduous teeth = 4 mo i.u – 3 mo of age for A, B teeth; 5 mo i.u. – 9 mo of age for C teeth.
- On permanent teeth = 3 –5 yrs age to 7 yrs age for 1, 2, 3 teeth.
- Oxytetracycline and doxycycline = cause less destruction
- Yellowish or brownish gray discoloration; it increases after exposure to light; fluorescence under UV light seen as bright yellow; mostly involves dentin; bleaching has less effect;

• **Angioneurotic edema** = aka **Quincke's edema**;

A biochemical abnormality = absence of inhibitor of C' 1 esterase enz from serum which then causes increased consumption of C'2 and C'4 and formation of kinin-like substances, which increase the vascular permeability and oedema.

Rx = antihistamine; eACA is an antifibrinolytic agent which blocks the activation of plasmin which then activates the complement cascade;

• **Drug allergy** = aka dermatitis medicamentosa (of skin)

And stomatitis medicamentosa (on oral m.m)

• **Contact dermatitis** = aka stomatitis and dermatitis venenata. = is due to Ag-Ab reactions at the site of contact, e.g. procaine; resin, etc.

• **Hairy tongue** = is due to elongation of filiform papillae = as a complication of antibiotics esp penicillin due to altered bacterial flora.

OCCUPATIONAL INJURIES

- As = necrosis of bone
- Bi = blue pigmentation of gingiva and oral m.m.
- Cr = necrosis of bone, ulceration of oral m.m.
- F = osteosclerosis
- Pb = blue-black pigmentation of gingiva
- Hg = ptyalism, osteomyelitis
- P = osteomyelitis, ulceration
- Aniline = blue coloration of lips/gingiva
- Benzene = blue coloration of lips
- Acids = decalcification of teeth
- CO, CO_2 = coloration of lips (cherry red, blue)
- Radium, x-rays = osteomyelitis; necrosis; xerostomia, etc.
- Actinic rays = carcinoma of lips
- Cu, Fe, Ni, Cr, etc. tobacco = staining of teeth

HEALING OF WOUNDS

- X-rays = in low doses, increase the healing and in high doses = decrease the healing
- Compounds containing free –SH groups = increase the healing rate of all amino acids, only METHIONINE has this group and which restores rate of healing to normal level in hypoproteinic groups.
- Vitamines = vit C = regulates collagen formation and ground substances. In scurvy, delayed healing is due to interference in formation of mucopolysaccharides which makes the cementing substances.
- Vit A = retards healing by affecting epithelial cells.
- Infections = wounds which are completely protected from bact. irritation heal more slowly than with infections.
- Hormonal factors = ACTH and cortisone interfere with healing — due to inhibition of fibroblastic and endothelial proliferation and inflammatory reaction. And delay in mesenchymal reaction.

- Diabetes mellitus = very slow to heal; retards the wound healing — due to disturbances in carbohydrate metabolism at cellular level in the local area of wound. Adding insulin = stimulates fibroblastic proliferation in tissue culture.
- Sutures = weaker wounds with non-absorbable sutures; lower rate of infections with monofilament suture than with multifilament sutures.
- Cyanoacrylates as chemical tissue adhesives = can be used in p.o moisture, hastens healing, is hemostatic and bacteriostatic.

Biopsy = is the removal of tissue from a living organism

- Excisional B. = total excision of small lesion.
- Incisional / diagnostic B. = for larger lesions
- Punch B
- Aspiration
- Exfoliative cytology = also helpful in diagnosis of other dis, e.g. herpes, pemphigus, etc.
- Surgical removal by cautery / high velocity cutting knife = but it dehydrates the tissues.

Surgical removal by scalpel = is best because it cleanly removes the tissues.

- Fixation of tissues = in 10 % formalin or 70% alcohol.

Always take normal tissue with pathologic tissue in the sample.

DRY SOCKET = aka localised acute alveolar osteomyelitis/alv. osteitis

Is a focal osteomyelitis – no suppuration

Very painful = pain appears 2–3 days after extractions

<u>Fibrinolysis of clot</u> by plasmin = is a major factor in pathogenesis.

Rx = local packs of ZOE, iosoform ec; aureomycin decreases incidence of decomposition of clots.

Myospherulosis = is a complication of healing of extraction wound in which there has been placed antibiotic ointment with a petrolatum base.

Trypsin = promotes healing by digesting necrotic tissues and debris and thus restains bacterial growth.

Fracture healing

- **External callus** = i.e. the new tissue formed around the outside of 2 fragments of the bone.
- **Internal callus** = i.e. the new tissue arising from the marrow cavity.
- **Anchoring** callus = on outside surface of the bone near the periosteum, it extends some distance away from the fracture. Produces spongy bone.
- **Sealing** callus = develops on the inside surface of the bone across the fractured end. It forms from endosteal proliferation. It fills the marrow space and goes out into the fracture site.
- **Bridging** callus = develops on the outside surface b/w the anchoring callus on the 2 ends. It is the only callus which is primarily cartilagenous.
- **Uniting** callus = forms b/w the ends of bones and b/w areas of other primary calluses that have formed on the 2 ends. It does not form until other types of callus are well developed, it forms by direct ossification.
- **Secondary** callus = is the mature bone which replaces the immature bone of primary callus. It is more heavily calcified and can be seen on R/G; can withstand active use, and pseudohaversian system is not formed uniformly.
- Periosteum is imp. for healing because its inner layer is osteogenic which gives rise to osteoblasts.

Replantation, i.e. placement of tooth with in same alveolar socket. Mature teeth with closed apices should be RCTed before it, while with open apices can be placed directly as chances of revascularisation are there. PDL should be preserved to avoid ankylosis, root resorption, etc.

Transposition, from one site to other site. It may be autogenous (BEST) or homogenous. Storage by freeze-drying (LYOPHILISATION) or by chemical coagulation by thiomersol/ merthiolate.

ORAL ASPECTS OF METABOLIC DISEASES

Optimal F intake = 0.05–0.07 mg /kg

Topical F gel = 10,000–12,300 ppm

F rinse 0.05% = 230 ppm

Cariostatic ions = F, P

Mildly cariostatic = Mo, V, Cu, Sr, B, Li, Au, Fe

Caries inert = Ba, Al, Ni, Pd, Ti

Caries promoting = Se, Mg, Cd, Pt, Pb, Si

Antiacidogenic effects = cheese; pyridoxin B_6; PO_4^-; Ca^- lactate; arginine rich peptides; and tea (amylase), fatty acids.

Calcium

- Membrane permeability, heart rhythm, neuromuscular excitability; blood clotting;
- Normal levels = 9–11 mg%
- If < 8 mg % = hyperirritability, tetany, carpopedal spasm
- If > 11 mg% = depressed nerve conductivity, muscle rigors;
- Blood level is controlled by parathyroid gland which is stimulated by low Ca^{++} levels and vice versa.
- Absorption = phytic acid makes insoluble Ca phytate and makes Ca non-available for absorption;
- Vit D increases Ca absorption from GIT
- Fat also helps in its absorption but in sprue, Ca is excreted with fats as soaps.
- Citrates help in absorption and calcification of bones.
- Decreased pH of GIT, e.g. hypo - / achlorhydria decrease absorption
- Lactose increase its retention.
- 80% Ca is excreted in feces.

PHOSPHORUS

- functions in phosphorylation in metabolism
- ATP for ms. contraction

- Coenzyme, e.g. pyridoxal phosphate
- Maintained by PTH, vit D, Pase activity
- Excreted mainly in urine

MAGNESIUM

- Participates in every phosphorylation mechanism.
- Excess excreted in urine
- Hyper- Mg esia = voluntary ms paralysis
- If it increases to 18–21 mg /dl = coma, death
- Deficiency = nm and vascular disturbances; enamel hypoplasia
- Mg deficient tetany = carpopedal spasm; + ve Chovstek's sign;

DYSTROPHIC CALCIFICATIONS= Ca salts deposited in dead or degenerating tissues; it is **most frequent type of pathologic calcifications**. It is most common in pulp of teeth esp of older patients; esp degenerated and inflammed pulps

Metastatic calcifications = Ca salts get precipitated in previously undamaged tissues; due to increased Ca in blood; esp in hyperparathyroidism in which Ca from bone goes to blood; in hypervitaminosis D; occurs in kidney/ lungs/ media of blood vessels;

Calcinosis = p.o. calcifications in or under the skin

Sodium

Mostly extracellular and in plasma

Maintains acid-base equilibrium and osmotic pressure

Normal levels = 160 mg %

Kidney is principal organ for excretion of water and salts

Aldosterone is released in case of excess loss of Na; which acts on renal tubules (DCT), to increase reabsorption and to conserve Na;

Addison's dis = salt depletion; extracellular water / Na are rapidly excreted by kidneys decrease in plasma Na conc; increase seurm K levels.

Potassium

Most of the K is intracellular;

90% of excreted K is eliminated in urine

urinary excretion is influenced by aldosterone which controls the active tubular secretion of K.

normal levels = 4 meq / litre of plasma.

Chlorine

Na , Cl are mimp, minerals constituents of the extracellular fluids. Cl is excreted primarily through kidneys. It activates the salivary amylase. Normal levels = 550–650 mg %

Trace elements

• Iodine = for formation of thyroid Hs; its deficiency leads to goitre; thyroxine formation is related to TYROSINE METABOLISM

• Copper = required for normal erythropoiesis; for Fe absorption which is mediated by ceruloplasmin. Its deficiency leads to anemia. Cu deficiency dis is ka **Menke's synd** (STEELY OR KINKY HAIR SYND).

• Iron = absorbed in upper part of duodenum; little excretion of Fe takes place either by GIT or kidneys, so it is ka ONE WAY SUBSTANCE.

Its deficiency leads to anemia; oesophageal webs in Plummer-Vinson syndrome

• Iron overload = leads to hemochromatosis;

Bantu's siderosis = by ingestion of home made beer fermented in iron-pots.

• Zinc = conc. of Zn in E and D is 0.02 % which is > in any other tissues.

Teeth of TB patients have higher conc of Zn.

Zn deficiency = lack of pubic / axillary hair; atrophic testes; retarded bone age; low levels of alkaline Pase enz.

• Mn = esp abundant in liver; necessary for activation of Pase; forms a part of enz arginase

• Co = found in vit. B_{12}; cyanocobalamine; used in Rx of pernicious anemia;

• Cr = role in carbohydrate and lipid metabolism; may facilitate insulin binding to cell membrane via a Cr-bridge, i.e. **potentiates insulin action**.

• Se = glutathione selenoenzyme is responsible for eliminating potentially harmful peroxides and free radicals.

• Protein deficiency = aka marasmus, e.g. in burns, hyperthyroidism, etc.

Kwarshiorkor = protein–energy deficiency in children; **caries free mouth;** decreased growth of jaws; delayed eruption; increased caries; decreased saliva volume.

Porphyria = overproduction of **uroporphyrin** and related substances;

Erythropoietic uroporphyria = congenital porphyria = excretion of red urine; red-brownish discoloration of teeth;

DISTURBANCES OF CARBOHYDRATE METABOLISM

Hurler 's synd; mucopolysaccharidosis - I; MPS–I H; gargoylism	Increase MPS secretions in urine; increased intracellular accumulation of chondroitin sulphate B and heparitin sulphate, C/F = corneal clouding; claw hands; saddle nose; enlarged tongue–open mouth; increased arch length and TYPICAL SPACING B/W TEETH; shortening and broading of mandible with prominent gonions; H/E = fibroblasts appear as clear cells or Gargoyl cells or Hurler's cells; Reilly bodies in circulating lymphocytes.
Lipoid proteinosis	Waxy nodules on skin, intracranial calcifications above the pituitary fossa; INA BILITY OF INFANT TO CRY AT BIRTH;
Hereditary fructose intolerance	Hypoglycemia; vomiting after ingestion of fructose containing foods; is due to deficiency of fructose – 1–phosphate aldolase enz.; decreased caries

DISTURBANCES IN LIPID METABOLISMS

a. non-reticuloendotheliosis = aka histiocytosis-X dis, e.g. Letterer-Siwe dis; = lymphomatous proliferation of poorly differentiated histiocytes;

   Hand-Schuller-Christian disease and eosinophilic granuloma = both are non-neoplastic reactions of well differentiated histiocytes; but EG is unifocal / solitary lesion.

b. lipid reticuloendotheliosis = due to specific lysosomal enz; e.g. Gaucher's dis; Niemann-Pick's dis.

Hand–Schuller – Christian disease/ multifocal EG	Both skeletal and extra-skeletal lesions; has chronic clinical course; TRIAD = punched out bone lesions; exophthalmos; diabetes insipidus; O/F = loss of supporting alveolar bone; advanced PD dis; failure of healing of extraction sockets; R/G = sharply outlined punched out lesions; severe alv. Bone loss; H/E = foam cells, i.e. cholesterol containing histiocytes.
Eosinophilic granuloma/ unifocal EG	Primarily, histiocytic proliferation. Only bony lesions; no intracellular accumulation of lipids; mainly skull and mandible; lesions are well demarcated and destructive; resembling cysts in R/G.
LS dis.	In infants < 3 yrs; diffuse destruction of mx/ md bone and so premature loss of teeth; histiocytes proliferation but no foam cells;
Gaucher's dis.	Defective lipid metabolism. Disturbance in glucosyl ceramide metabolism; lipid filled histiocytes ka GAUCHER'S CELLS; are pathognomonic; found in liver; spleen; bone marrow, etc.; they have wrinkled/ *crumpled silk cytoplasm*. Kerasin is deposited in RE cells.

Disturbances in Lipid Metabolisms (*Contd.*)

Niemann-Pick dis.	Disturbance of sphingomyelin metab.; pathognomonic cells are +nt ka Niemann-Pick cells in RE system

VITAMINS

Provitamins are vitamins which occur in natural sources in inactive form and become active only in the animal.

Fat soluble = A, D, E, K

Water soluble = B, C

Vitamin A	Regulates epithelial differentiation; In deficiency = keratinising metaplasia of epithelial cells; **Epithelial invasion of pulpal tissue** is a characteristic feature. Atypical dentin lacking tubular arrangement. <u>Increased caries susceptibility</u> due to change in salivary glands functions. PD infections and micro-abscess formations. Deficiency = night blindness; xerophthalmia; keratomalacia; Hypervitaminosis A = pronounced periosteal thickening; but no change in salivary glands functions.
Vitamin D	Cholecalciferol; controls Ca^{++} ions conc. It exerts its major influence by combining with non- histone proteins in the nuclei of intestinal epith cells; Hypervitaminosis D → hypercalcemia Hypovitaminosis D → sec. hyperparathyroidism; PTH levels increase and serum Ca ions level are maintained at the expense of bone; serum PO_4 ions levels decrease due to PTH effect of renal excretion of PO_4 ions.

Vitamins (*Contd.*)

	Serum alk P ase levels increase due to bone's attempt at repair;
Vit D deficient rickets	Hypomineralised bone matrix, i.e. a failure of endochondral calcification. C/F = ms weak; atony; cessation of calcification of epiphyseal disks → chondroblasts get nutrition and do not die; keep on growing and multiplying → irregular increased width of disk. Bowing of legs due to hypocalcified bones unable to bear the weight. O/F = abnormal E and D dev; delayed eruption; higher caries index; increased interglobular dentin; Diet high in **phytate (**it binds with available diet-Ca^{++}**)** leads to bony deformities; ERGOCALCIFEROL added to milk helps in prevention of rickets;
Osteomalacia/adult rickets	Only flat bones and diaphysis of long bones are affected; C/F = softening, distortion and FRACTURE OF bones; R/G = asymmetric deformities of all stress bearing bones; longitudinal hairline fractures in long bones;
Vit D resistant rickets	Aka **refractory rickets** or **phosphate diabetes**; Hypophosphatemia; hyperphosphaturia; Does not respond to usual doses of vit D; **Retarded dental eruption**; **Pulp horns elongated** often reaching DEJ; PA involvement of grossly normal appearing deciduous or permanent teeth and dev. of multiple gingival fistulas; Lamina dura poorly defined/irregular/abnormal alveolar bone/cementum; H/E = failure of bone salts to be deposited in cartilage matrix;

Vitamins (*Contd.*)

	Broad zone b/w shaft and cartilage cells = ka RACHITIC METAPHYSIS;
Renal rickets	Renal osteodystrophy; painful-crippling bone dis. It is due to inability of kidneys to synthesise 1-alpha-hydroxylase and convert 25-hydroxycholecalciferol to the active form of vit D; DRAMATIC increase in fecal Ca excretion and negative N_2 balance; Sec. Hyperparathyroidism may cause osteitis fibrosis cystica;
Hypophosphatasia	Aka hypophosphatasemia; Due to deficiency of enz. Alk. Pase; excretion of phospho-ethanol- amine in urine; O/F = **loosening and premature loss of deciduous teeth** esp incisors; Hypocalcified teeth; LARGE PULP CHAMBERS; alv. bone loss; ABSENCE OF CEMENTUM on teeth due to failure of cemento-genesis → so no sound functional attachment of tooth to bone by PDL; so early loss of primary teeth
Vitamin E; tocopherol	**Antioxidant** = plays role in free radical damage protection; Main function is to prevent peroxidation of PUFA. Deficiency causes impaired fetal-maternal vascular relation.
Vitamin K	Transported to liver via lymph chylomicrons; Helps in synth of 2, 7, 9, 10 clotting factors in liver esp prothrombin, i.e. factor 2. **Dicoumarol** = is vit. K antagonist. Most common oral feature of vit. K def. = gingival bleeding;
Vitamin C; ascorbic acid; hexuronic acid	Most animals are capable of synthesising their own vit C except monkey, human, guinea pigs because they are unable to convert L-gluconolactone to L–ascorbic acid; Roles = reqd for H-transfer, maintenance of intra

Vitamins (*Contd.*)

	cellular oxidation reduction potential; antioxidant; helps Fe uptake from GIT; involved in formation of folinic acid Reqd in hydroxylation of proline in collagen synthesis. Normal dev of ground substances in bone, dentin, other CTs, etc. Deficiency = scurvy; atrophy and disorganisation of odontoblasts and irregular dentin formation;
Scurvy	Hemorrhage in PDL; loss of bone; loosening of teeth and exfoliation; foul breath of fusospirochetal organisms; healing is delayed as fibroblasts fail to produce collagen. Subperiosteal hemorrhage is common. **Scorbutic lattice** = a wide zone of calcified but non-ossified matrix in metaphysis due to continuous proliferation of cartilage cells and deposition of calcified salts in b/w the columns, so fragility of bones occurs; **Trummerfeld zone** = is the region of complete disintegration; here, fracture of calcified matrix occurs which is a classic picture of scurvy; **Gerustmark** = area below trummerfeld zone is free of hemato-poietic cells and is made of CT cells.
Vitamin B complex	Animal cells are incapable of synthesising all vitamins B except nicotinic acid and choline. Except vit B_{12}, no other vit B is stored in tissues of body but get excreted in urine; found in meat, etc. Thiamine; B_1 def = **beri beri**; multiple neuritis, CHF; generalised edema; Riboflavin B_2 = is a constituent of coenz FMN and FAD which are essential to oxidative enz systems utilising electron transport system; Riboflavin def = common in children who **do not drink milk**;

Vitamins (*Contd.*)

Riboflavin def	C/F = glossitis + dermatitis + ocular changes; Glossitis = filiform papillae atrophic; fungiform papillae become engorged/mushroom shaped = **granular tongue; magenta colored** Tongue may be smooth; glazed due to atrophy of all papilae
Niacin	Niacin → nicotinic acid amide → forms coenz I (NAD); and coenz II (NADP); **tryptophan** gives rise to nicotinic acid in p.o. of **pyridoxal-5-phosphate**. Deficiency = PELLAGRA, i.e. rough skin; S/S = 4 ***D***'s, i.e. ***d***iarrhoea, ***d***ementia; ***d***ermatitis and ***d***eath; Tongue = burning sensation; swelling; dental indentation; scalded mouth, red and painful; superimposed ANUG
Pantothenic acid	Is a constituent of coenzyme A
Pyridoxine B_6	Is a complex of 3 substances = pyridoxine + pyridoxal + pyridoxamine; involved in tryptophan metabolism; p.o. xanthurenic acid in urine = is a biologic test for B_6 deficiency.
Choline	Imp constituent of lecithine, sphingomyelin and Ach; Need for choline depends on their sources of methyl group in diet esp **methionine;** <u>methionine is precursor of choline</u>. Diets high in choline, Methionine and proteins is used for Rx of fatty liver and cirrhosis esp in chronic alcoholics
Folic acid	Primary function = transfer of one-C moieties; Also reqd in purine synthesis; Synth of DNA is impossible in absence of folic acid.
Folic acid def	C/ F = Glossitis + diarrhoea + macrocytic anemia; Filiform papillae are first to disappear; Also seen in Rx of leukemia with **aminopterin.**

Vitamins (*Contd.*)

	Aminopterin interferes with conversion of FA to folinic acid; so folic acid is given for Rx of aminopterin toxicity.
Vitamin B_{12}	Cyanocobalamine; Antipernicious factor; High doses can be used for Rx of = trigeminal neuralgia

DISTURBANCES OF HORMONE METABOLISM

Pituitary gland	Anterior lobe = derived from Rathke's pouch; epithelial in origin; glandular in structure; 6 hormones. It is also = ketogenic; anti-insulin; diabetogenic; pancreatotropic activity. Posterior lobe = dev from floor of 3rd ventricle; composed of neural tissues; has three actions = vasoconstrictor; oxytocic; antiduretic. Removal of pituitary gland = leads to atrophy of all endothelial glands except parathyroid.
Decreased pituitary hormones	Delays eruption of teeth; Thickening of dentinal walls at the expense of pulp chambers; Amelogenesis directly depends on pit. H; but dentino- / cemento- can proceed at decreased rate without pit. H. Thyroxin stimulates eruptive movement and tooth size, but little effect on alveolar growth;
Hypopituitarism	Causes DWARFISM; delayed eruption; over-retained teeth; small dental arch and M.O.; smaller roots; dev. of maxilla is not as retarded as mandible (so CLASS II);
Simmond's dis	Hypopituitarism in adults due to infarcts of gland = ka panhypopituitarism;

Disturbances of Hormone Metabolism (*Contd.*)

	Skin has atrophic changes, immobile expressions;
Hyperpituitarism	Causes GIGANTISM in infants and ACROMEGALY in adults; If increases before closure of epiphysis of long bones = gigantism If increases after closure of epiphysis of long bones = acromegaly. Tongue size is increased; mandible increase in size (CLASS III); DIABETES also occurs in patients.
Thyroid H	Causes increased uptake of O_2 by body and controls many physiological functions;
Calcitonin	Secreted by C-cells; is responsive to hypercalcemia; acts to decrease plasma Ca^{-}-level; inhibits resorption of bone minerals.
Hypothyroidism	♦ cretinism = in infants; juvenile myxedema = in children; ♦ myxedema = in adults; **Cretinism** = mental def; growth retardation; generalised oedema; mandibular underdevelop + maxillary overdevelop = CLASS II; Sweat glands atrophic so dry skin; Tongue = size increases due to edema, so protrude and **spacing.** Teeth = retarded eruption; over-retained deciduous teeth; Myxedema = swelling; increased blood protein conc.; tongue edematous / large which interferes with speech;
Hyperthyroidism; **Grave's dis**	Increased BMR; moist skin; urinary excretion of I2 decreases; Premature fall of deciduous teeth; Alveolar atrophy in advanced cases;

Disturbances of Hormone Metabolism (*Contd.*)

	Accelerated eruption of permanent teeth; very poor dental patients; Increased susceptibility to Adr; hypertension; Wide eyes stairing; anxious looks;
Primary hyper-parathyroidism	Increased amount of PTH; PTH has no cysteine; Hypercalcemia and poor ms tone; decreased nm excitability; C/F = pathologic fractures may be the first S/S. Urinary tract stone; giant cell tumors or a cyst of jaw; Generalised osteoporosis = loss of P and Ca; Pseudocyst formation = due to resorption of new bone formed. Malocclusion = sudden drifting of teeth; R/G = R/L sharply defined round / oval areas which may be lobulated (D/D = ameloblastoma) Small cystic areas in U/L jaws, skull (D/D = multiple myeloma; eosinophilic granuloma) **Ground glass appearance.** Lamina dura around the teeth may be partially lost. H/E = mimp feature = **osteoclastic resorption of trabeculae of spongiosa** and along the blood vessels in haversian system of cortex. Osteoclastomas develop = (D/D = central giant cell granuloma) Increased serum Ca^{++} levels (normal = 9–12 mg %) Rx = excision of gland.
Secondary hyper-parathyroidism	Aka **von-Recklinghausen's dis of bones;** Develop due to chronic/ end - stage renal disease;

Disturbances of Hormone Metabolism (*Contd.*)

	Loss of lamina dura; increase serum alk Pase; brown tumors develop
Hypo-parathyroidism	Low conc of serum Ca; high conc of serum P; If Ca is < 7–8 mg % = increased nm excit-ability If Ca is < 5–6 mg % = tetany; carpopedal spasm; Hypoplasia of teeth; chronic candidiasis is present and precedes hypocalcemia and it may cause hypoparath. by an immune response
Pseudo hypo-parathyroidism	The parathyroid extract has little/ no effect in correcting the hypocalcemia.
ADRENALS	Adrenal cortex = plays the essential role in maintaining life. Adrenal medulla = Adr and N-Adr has effects like sympathetic nervous system stimulation. Increased Adr in body = increases BMR by its effect on liver and on carbohyd metabolism rather on thyroid gland; Adr = causes constriction of arterioles and capillaries of skin; m.m; abdominal viscera; dilatation of vessels of skeletal and heart ms; NET RESULT = increase in BP due to a sufficient vasoconstriction of end-capillaries and arterioles of skin, etc. Under controlled conditions = Adr acts as an overall vasodilator and a powerful cardiac stimulant, while N Adr as overall vasocons.
Waterhouse – Friderichsen syndr.	Acute insufficiency of adr. Cortex; septicemia, purpura; and petechiae; death within 2–3 days;

Disturbances of Hormone Metabolism (*Contd.*)

Addison's dis	Chronic insufficiency of adr cortex; C/F = bronzing of skin; pigmentation of m.m, (it may be first sign of dis, spreading on lips, gingiva, etc.) H/E = acanthosis with silver +ve granules in cells of Str. germinativum. Patient carries BLUE WARNING CARD (as an indication on systemic steroid Rx)
Hyperfunction of adrenal gland	Adrenogenital synd; and **Cushing's synd;** Cushing dis = Cushing synd + spontaneous bilateral adrenal hyperplasia. S/S = fat deposition on upper part of body; mooning of face; buffalo hump; glycosuria not controlled by insulin; O/F = osteoporosis; premature cessation of epiphyseal growth.
Stress and adaptation synd	Cortisone interferes with formation of granulation tissues, fibroblast proliferation and wound healing, so SURGERY IS HAZARDOUS IN hyperadrenocorticism.
Diabetes mellitus	Significant thickening of basement membrane of gingival vessels; decrease tissue resistance to infections; PD abscess; even minor surgery is C/I in DM.
Progeria	Aka **Hutchinson-Gilford syndrome**; prematurely old; dwarfism and premature senility. C/F = beak like nose; hypoplastic mandible; coxa valga is a constant feature; early death. O/F = delayed dental eruption; increased formation of irregular dentin;

DISEASES OF NERVOUS TISSUES

Trigeminal neuralgia; tic-douloureux; Fothergill's dis; trifacial neuralgia	Etio = circulatory insufficiency or reflex vasocons of Gasserian ganglion. Attack provoked by vasocons; relieved by vasodilators Also found in patients with multiple sclerosis; C/F = right side; unilateral; seldom crosses the midline; trigger zones. Rx = injection of alcohol; carbamazepine; microsurgical decompression of trigeminal root (BEST) D/D = migraine; migrainous neuralgia (Horton's synd;) but it has no trigger zone and persists for hours.
tic-douloureux;	When patient suffers from spasmodic contraction of facial ms.
Costen's synd	Increased size of styloid process
Trotter's synd	Nasopharyngeal tumor + pain in lower jaw, tongue, side of head + middle ear deafness.+ defective mobility of soft palate + trismus of internal pterygoid ms. Its main cause is involvement of mandibular N in foramen ovale
Herpes zoster of 5th nerve	Ka post-herpetic neuralgia = pain usually involves the ophthalmic div of 5th N.
Raeder's synd ; paratrigeminal synd	Pain in the area of 5th N distribution + ocular sympathetic paralysis. No change in sweating activity (as cp to Horner's synd)
Horton's synd; sphenopalatine neuralgia; vidian n. neuralgia;	Etio = due to vasodilation of internal maxillary A. (of ECA); C/F = no trigger zones; aka **alarm clock headache** (as it occurs at the same time of the day); **Rx** = cocainization/alcohol inj. in spheno-

Diseases of Nervous Tissues (*Contd.*)

lower half headache; cluster headache	palatine ganglion. Ergotamine &/or methysergide (antiserotonin agent) = for total relief; Vidian n = n. of pterygoid canal = gr. Petrosal n + deep petrosal n.
Orolingual paresthesia	Glossodynia = painful tongue; glossopyrosis = burning tongue.
Frey's/ Dupuy's/ auriculotemporal syndrome/ gustatory sweating	Etio = due to damage to auriculotemporal n & subsequent re-innervation of sweat glands by p-symp salivary fibres. C/F = sweating of involved side of face esp temporal area during eating; also may be evoked by parentral admn of PILOCARPINE and eliminated by atropine or by procaine block to auriculotemporal N. **Crocodile tears** = profuse lacrimation while eating is due to salivary-lacrimal reflex arc development.
Bell's palsy; facial paralysis	Etio = ischemia of nerve near the stylomandibular foramen; inj. Of LA in capsule of parotid gland. C/F = facial ms actions not possible; expressionless / mask like face; taste sensation of anterior 3rd tongue altered. Rx = nicotinic acid; vasodilator drugs; decompression of nerve.
Melkersson-Rosenthal synd Glossopharyngeal neuralgia	Bell's palsy + facial edema + cheilitis granulomatosa + fissured tongue/ lingua plicata. Sharp shooting pain in ear, pharynx, nasopharynx, tonsil or posterior part of tongue. Trigger zone present in post. Oropharynx/ tonsillar fossa.
Multiple sclerosis/	Is a demyelinating dis affecting mainly the white matter of CNS;

Diseases of Nervous Tissues (*Contd.*)

disseminated sclerosis	Etio = due to scattered venous thrombi; or as allergic hypersensitivity due to Ag-Ab reacations. Patients have increased gamma-globulin conc in CSF; CHARCOT'S TRIAD = intention tremors + nystagmus + dysartheria/scanning speech.
Orofacial dyskinesia	Etio = a complication of phenothiazine (antipsychotic) Rx. Or due to disruption of dental proprioception (as in edentulous patients as they have no PDL).
Menier's dis	Deafness + tinnitus + vertigo; Deafness = is inner ear deafness of conductive type; there is dilatation of endolymphatic spaces of labyrinth with the absence of an inflammatory reaction. Rx = vasodilators, e.g. histamine; niacin (nicotinic acid)
Migraine	Is a discharge of autonomic centers in forebrain leading to constriction in parts of cerebral arterial tree. **Prodromal phase**/pre-headache phenomenon is present. Mainly unilateral Rx = ergotamine; methysergide, nor-epinephrine
Temporal arteritis; giant cell arteritis	Is atypical migraine; due to immunologic reaction to elastic lamina of As; ESR is markedly raised. Rx = corticosteroids
Causalgia	Pain after injury to or sectioning of peripheral sensory N.

Diseases of Nervous Tissues (*Contd.*)

	Usually follows the extraction of multirooted teeth. • pain/attack may be elicited not only by actual touch stimulation but also by emotional disturbances. • Rx = resection of ns in retrogasserian region
Atypical facial pain / facial causalgia	Pain in the areas supplied by 5th and 9th cranial nerves and 2nd and 3rd cervical nerves. Distribution of pain is unanatomic, MAY CROSS MIDLINE. No trigger zone;
Eagle's synd	Elongation of styloid process or ossification of stylohyoid lig. Pain along the distribution of ECA/ICA and pharyngeal pain. Carotid A synd = styloid process pressing vs ICA/ECA.
Horner's synd/ sympathetic ophthalmoplegia	Triad = miosis + ptosis + anhidrosis and vasodilation over the face. Esp pregang. fibres in anterior spinal roots to the symp chain in the low cervical and high thoracic area are involved.
Jaw winking synd/Marcus Gunn phenomenon	Pterygoid levator synkinesis; Congenital unilateral ptosis with rapid elevation of ptotic eyelid occurring on the movement of mandible to the contralateral side.
Marin-Amat synd	Inverted Marcus Gunn phenomenon; seen after peripheral facial paralysis; C/F = eye closes automatically when patient opens his mouth fully and forcibly and tears may flow.

DISEASES OF MUSCLES

Dystrophic myotonia	*Myotonia is failure of ms relaxation after cessation of voluntary contraction.* Atrophy of ms; pt has myopathic facies and **swan neck appearance**; recurrent TMJ dislocation; **testicular dystrophy**;
Congenital myotonia; Thomsen's dis	Myotonia ass. with hypertrophy of ms, affects all skeletal ms esp of lower limb; so inability of child to walk or stand; ms show prolonged contraction and delay in relaxation. HERCULEAN APPEARANCE of the patient. Attack prompted by sudden movements, e.g. sneezing.
Paramyotonia	Not ass. with ms wasting; cramping attacks are prompted by COLD; face has **mask like appearance**;
Hypotonia	Bodies of infants hang limply with inability to sit, stand or walk; ka **floppy infant synd;**
Myasthenia gravis	Progressive **weakness of skeletal ms** esp those innervated by cranial ns; defective nm transmission (as after inj of curare); fault is in **acetylcholine mechanism**; is due to thymus gland exhibiting lymphoid follicular hyperplasia; weak facial ms giving sorrowful appearance; Therapeutic **diagnosis** = I/M inj of physostigmine (anticholinesterase)
Dermatomyositis	Symmetrical involvement of ms with stiffness/ weakness; **calcinosis cutis** i.e. skin lesions calcify to form CaCO3 nodules with a foreign body reaction; **calcinosis universalis** i.e. if calcified masses are through the soft tissues; CREATINURIA is a constant finding.
Generalised/ progressive	Affects interstitial tissue of ms; tendons; ligaments; slowly entire ms get transformed

Diseases of Muscles (*Contd.*)

myositis ossificans	in bone resulting in limitation of movements; patient becomes a **rigid organism** ka PETRIFIED MAN.
Traumatic myositis ossificans	Aka Ossifying hematome, e.g. RIDER'S BONE, i.e. thigh adductor ms of horse riders; DRILL/EXERCISE BONE, i.e. deltoid/pectoral region of soldiers; R/G = feathery type calcification in ms.
Mobius synd	Congenital facial diplegia; deficient dev of cranial ms; + facial diplegia + bilateral paralysis of ocular ms esp ABDUCENS. C/F = failure to close the eyes during sleep of child;

APPENDICES

Normal Blood Values

	Males	Females	
RBCs count	4.5–6.5 millions/c.mm average = 5.5	3.8– 5.8 millions c.mm; average = 4.8	
Half-life of RBC			120 days
Hb	14–18 gm %	12–16 gm %	
Hematocrit/ PCV	45 % ; 40–54 %	37–47 %	
ESR in 1 hr; Wintrobe's method	0–6.5 mm	0–15 mm, i.e. more in females	

Appendices (*Contd.*)

	Males	**Females**	
ESR in 1 hr by Westergren's method	0–6 mm = normal; 7–20 mm = doubtful; > 20 mm = abnormal.		
MCV	80–90 cu. micron		
MCH	30 pg / 27–32 micro-micro gm.		
MCHC	30–35 % (33 gm/100ml of packed cells)		
TLC	4,000–11,000/ c.mm		
Neutrophils	50–70 %		
Lymphocytes	20–30 %		
Monocytes	2–8 %		
Eosinophils	1–4 %		
Basophils	0–1 %, i.e. least in number.		
Platelets	1.5–4 lacs /c.mm		
BT	< 5 min, Duke's method upto 11 min., ivy method		
CT	2.5–5 min, Kruse and Moses method; 1–7 min; capillary tube method; 5–10 min; Lee and White method		

Appendices (Contd.)

	Males	**Females**	
PT	10–20 sec; Quick method		
Clot retraction time	Begins at 1–6 hrs; completed in 24 hrs		
Capillary fragility by tourniquet test	+ve if > 10 petechiae/ inch circle		
Heterophile Abs	Below 1 : 56 dilution		

Incidence of Blood Groups

- Group O = 40 %
- A = 45 %
- B = 12 %
- AB = 4%
- Rh + = 85 %
- Rh - = 15%
- A+ ve = maximum

Values of Urine

Specific gravity	1.015–1.025	Cl	9.0 gm/lt
Volume / 24 hrs	1500 ml	Na	4 "
PH	Slightly acidic	K	2 "
Water	95 % of total volume	P	2 "
Urea	15–25 gm/litre	S	1.5 "
Uric acid	0.4–0.6 gm/lt	Ca. Mg	0.2 "
Creatinine	0.8–1.5 gm/lt		
Ammonia	0.6 gm/lt		

Serum Biochemical Values

SGOT	10–35 iu/l	
SGPT	10–40 iu/l	
Alk P ase	40–100 iu/l	
Acid Pase	0.1–0.4 iu/l	
Ascorbic acid	0.4–1.0 mg/dl	
Bilirubin	0.3–1.0 mg/dl	
Calcium / total	8.5–10.5 mg /dl	70–90 % of ingested calcium is excreted in feces and 10–30% in urine.
Creatinine	0.6–1.7 mg/dl	
Creatinine clearance	90–130 ml/ min	
Glucose/ fasting	70–110 mg %	
Glucose PP	< 140 mg%	
Glucose, whole blood	60–90 mg %	
Glucose, serum	70–105 mg %	
Iron binding capacity/ saturation	14–47 %	
Total serum proteins	6.2–8.2 gm %	
Albumin	3.6–4.7 gm %	
Globulin	2.4–3.7 gm %	
A:G ratio	1.5–2.5 : 1	
Urea	15–40 mg %	
Total cholesterol	120–260 mg %	

Miscellaneous Values

Total body fluid	50–70 % of body wt.
Intracellular fluid	30–40 %
Extracellular	20–30 %
BMR	– 15 % to + 15 %
Bilirubin / van den Bergh	Direct = 0–0.2 Total = 0.1–1.0
Volume of blood	70–100 cc/kg body wt
Volume of plasma	35–50 cc / kg wt
PH of blood	7.3–7.5
H^+ conc in blood	7.3–7.5

Syndromes

Addison's anemia	Aka pernicious/Biermer anemia; deficiency of intrinsic and extrinsic factors; triad = generalized weakness + sore painful tongue + numbness/ tingling of extremities
Addison's dis	Chronic insufficiency of adrenal cortex; bronzing of skin; pigmentation of m.m
Albright's synd	Polyostotic fibrous dysplasia + skin pigmentation + endocrine disturbances
Aldrich's synd	Thrombocytopenic purpura + eczema + susceptibility to infections
Apert synd	Syndactyly with Crouzon's disease
Ascher's synd	Acquired double lip + blepharochalasis + non toxic thyroid enlargement
Beckwith's hypoglycemic synd	Macroglossia + neonatal hypoglycemia + umbilical hernia, etc.

Syndromes (*Contd.*)

Behcet's synd	Recurrent oral ulcers; recurrent genital ulcers; ocular inflammation
Bowen dis	Intraepith carcinoma on skin esp in patients on As Rx.
Chediak-Higashi synd	Oculocutaneous albinism + phtophobia + nystagmus + recurrent infections
Costen's synd	Impaired hearing + tinnitus + otalgia + dizziness + headache, burning throat + TMJ problems, etc.
Cowden's synd	Facial trichilemmomas + oral papillomatous lesions. It is considered cutaneous marker of breast cancer. Multiple hamartomas + neoplasia synd
Crest synd	Calcinosis cutis; Raynaud's phenomenon; esophageal dysfunction; sclerodactyly; telangiectasia
Crohn' s dis	Regional enteritis / ileitis
Cushing dis	Cushing syndrome Associated with spontaneous bilateral adrenal hyperplasia
Cushing synd	Hyperfunction of adrenal gland
Darrier's dis	Verrucous, foul smelling masses + keratotic thickening of skin of palm, etc.; corps ronds and grains +nt.
Donath Seifert adeno Ca.	Epithelial-myoepithelial ca. of intercalated duct origin
Eagle synd	Elongation of styloid process or ossification of SH lig; dysphagia; otalgia; glossodynia, etc.
Ehler's Danlos synd	Hyperextensibility of joints + fragile skin + defective healing + excessive bruising; suturing not possible

Syndromes (*Contd.*)

Every's synd	It is associated with erupting third molar
Fanconi's synd	Familial aplastic anemia + microcephaly + hypogenitalism + bone abnormalities + brown pigmentation of skin
Gardener's synd	Multiple polyposis of large intestine + osteomas of bones + multiple epidermoid or sebaceous cysts + dermoid tumors, impacted supernumerary and permanent teeth
Goldenhar synd	Hemifacial microsomia aka oculoauriculovertebral synd
Grinspan synd	Lichen planus; hyperglycemia; hypertension
Heck's dis	Focal epith hyperplasia; esp on lower lip
Horner's synd	Miosis + ptosis + anhydrosis; damage of sympath. Pathways
Hurler's synd	Large head + typical facial features + large tongue + open mouth + corneal clouding + claw hands, etc.
Melkersson-Rosenthal synd	Cheilitis granulomatosa + facial paralysis (bilateral) + scrotal tongue
Plummer-Vinson synd	Pallor of skin + painful tongue + dysphagia with esophageal strictures
Reiter's synd	Tetrad = Urethritis; arthritis; conjunctivitis; mucocutaneous lesions
Rubeinstein-Taybi synd	Talon cusp + retarded development + delayed descent of testes, etc.
Sipple synd	Mucosal neuromas; medullary carcinoma of thyroid; pheochromocytoma
Vander Woud's synd	Pits of lower lip; cleft of palate
Vincent's infection	ANUG

Syndromes (*Contd.*)

Waterhouse-Friderichsen synd	Acute adrenal cortical insufficiency associated with ACUTE SEPTICEMIA
Goltz-Gorlin synd	Focal dermal hypoplasia + herniation of subcutaneous tissues + skin atrophy + syn-/polydactyly + notched alae + asymmetrical ears, etc.
Gorlin-Goltz synd	Basal cell nevi + OKC + bifid ribs + neurologic and eye abnormalities, etc.
Peutz jegher synd	Melanin pigmentation + intestinal polyposis; GI cancers.
Rendu-Osler-Weber dis	Spider like telengiectasis + epistaxis; primary intrinsic defectin endothelial cells
Sturge-Weber dis	Venous angiomas (esp in skin supplied by 5th nerve) + intracranial calcifications + neurologic manifestations
Higoumenaki's sign	Irregular thickening of sternoclavicular part of clavicle in congenital syphilis

Most Common Sites / Occurrence

Adenomatoid odontogenic tumor	Maxillary canine region
Ameloblastoma	Mand. Molar/ ramus area
Basal cell Ca.	Middle 3rd of face on skin; ka rodent ulcer
Bohn's nodules	Along the junction of hard and soft palate
Branchial cleft cyst	Lateral aspect of neck; along the anterior border of SCM m.
Complex Composite odontoma	Posterior jaws

Most Common Sites / Occurrence (*Contd.*)

Compound Composite odontoma	Anterior maxilla region
Dens evaginatus	B/w buccal and lingual cusp of premolars
Dens in dente	Permanent U lateral incisors
Dentigerous cyst	Mand/ max 3rd molar area and max canine area (the most common sites of impaction)
Enameloma	Near the bi- / trifurcation of roots of teeth near CEJ
Epstein pearls	Along the median raphe of hard palate
Fordyce's granules	Bilaterally on buccal mucosa of cheeks opposite the molars
Globulomaxillary cyst	B/W maxillary lateral incisor and canines
Intraoral ca	Tongue
Keratoacanthoma	Lips
Leukoplakia	Buccal mucosa
Most rapid metastasising tumor	African/ Burkitt jaw lymphoma
Oral carcinoma	Lips
Papilloma	Tongue
Pindborg's tumor	Associated with unerupted or impacted tooth?
Pleomorphic adenoma	Parotid gland
Primordial cyst	Dev. in place of permanent tooth; so retained deciduous tooth; as permanent tooth is absent
Static bone cyst	B/w mand canal and inferior border of mandible, i.e. below the mand canal

Most Common Sites / Occurrence (*Contd.*)

Talon cusp	U/L permanent incisors on lingual surface
Taurodontism	Permanent/ deciduous molars
Thyroglossal cyst	In midline; at any site from tongue to the thyroid gland

Most Common

2nd Most common impacted tooth	Permanent. Max canines
Ankylosis is most common in which primary tooth	Primary. Mand 2nd molar
Anomalous accessional permanent tooth	3rd molars
Anomalous succesional tooth	Max 2
Arch most affected by caries	Maxillary
Benign oral cancer	Fibroma
Bifid mand canal	In neurofibromatosis
Blood group in India	O+
Blood group in world	A+
Cleft lip	Unilateral complete
Fissural cyst	Median anterior palatine cyst
Greatest variation in onset of mineralisation in the initial appearance on R/G	Mand 5
Highest degree of viability wrt initiation of tooth bud	Mand 2nd premolar
Least affected by caries	Mand. 1 and 2; permanent
Mandibular most common malposed tooth due to space loss	2nd premolar

Most Common

Malignant tumor of major salivary glands	Adenocarcinoma
Metastatic lesion to jaw bones is from the primary tumor located in	Breast
Missing permanent teeth	3rd molar > mand 5> max 2 > max 5 > mand 1
Missing primary teeth	Max B > maxillary A > D
Most common caries of old age	Root surface;
Most common impacted tooth	Third molars
Most common missing tooth next to 3rd molar	2nd premolar
Nevus	Intradermal
Odontogenic cyst	Radicular cyst
Odontogenic tumor	Ameloblastic fibroma/ compound odontoma
Retained primary teeth	Mand E
Site of SCC	Lower lip near mucocutaneous junction
Supernum primary tooth	Max lateral
Supernumerary tooth	Mesiodens > distomolar, etc.
Surface most affected by caries	Occlusal surface
Tooth most affected by caries	Mand 6
Tumor of oral mucosa	SCC
Tumor of parotid gland	Pleomorphic adenoma
Upper most common crowded tooth	Permanent max canine
Used brushing tech	Scrub tech
Used disclosing agent	Erythrosin

18

MCQs in Oral Pathology

1. **Oral radiographs of a patient with scleroderma would show:**
   A. A "sun-ray" appearance of the bone
   B. An obscure lamina dura
   C. An abnormal widening of the periodontal ligament
   D. Vertical bone loss

2. **Which of the following soft tissue tumors is most likely to be found over the mental foramen in an edentulous patient?**
   A. Traumatic neuroma
   B. Neurilemoma (Schwannoma)
   C. Neurofibroma
   D. Neuroblastoma

3. **All of the following conditions demonstrate pigmentation of the intraoral mucous membranes except:**
   A. Addison's disease
   B. Albright syndrome
   C. Cushing syndrome
   D. Peutz-Jeghers syndrome

4. **Which cyst listed below is found in place of a tooth rather than directly associated with one?**
   A. Residual cyst
   B. Traumatic bone cyst
   C. Primordial cyst
   D. Periodontal cyst

5. **The etiology of verruciform xanthoma is:**
   A. Bacterial
   B. Viral
   C. Fungal
   D. Unknown

6. **All of the following are characteristics of Sjogren's syndrome except:**
   A. Rheumatoid arthritis
   B. Nephrosclerosis
   C. Xerostomia (dry mouth)
   D. Keratoconjunctivitis sicca (dryness of the eyes)

7. **Traumatic bone cysts are non-cysts often found in:**
   A. Infants
   B. Teenagers
   C. Middle aged adults
   D. Elderly people

8. **Which odontogenic tumor listed below has a high rate of recurrence if it is inadequately treated?**
   A. Odonotogenic myxoma
   B. Odontogenic fibroma
   C. Squamous cell carcinoma
   D. Pleomorphic adenoma

9. **Which of the following odontogenic cysts is always associated with the crown of an unerupted or developing tooth?**
   A. Lateral periodontal cyst
   B. Dentigerous cyst
   C. Odontogenic keratocyst
   D. Lateral Periodontal cyst

10. **The most common site in the oral cavity for a lymphangioma is the:**
    A. Palate
    B. Tonsils
    C. Floor of the mouth
    D. Tongue

11. The most common site for pyogenic granuloma to occur is:
A. The palate
B. The mucogingival junction
C. The interdental gingiva
D. The tongue

12. Which of the following tumors is also called the Pindborg tumor?
A. Adenomatoid odontogenic tumor
B. Calcifying epithelial odontogenic tumor
C. Squamous odontogenic tumor
D. Pleomorphic adenoma

13. The most frequently encountered intraoral benign neoplasm of connective tissue origin is:
A. A papilloma
B. A fibroma
C. A lipoma
D. A nodular melanoma

14. Which odontogenic tumor listed below usually affects males under the age of 25 years old?
A. Benign cementoblastoma
B. Gigantiform cementoma
C. Ameloblastoma
D. Squamous cell carcinoma

15. A dental granuloma and a radicular cyst can be differentiated:
A. Based on symptoms
B. Radiographically
C. Histologically
D. By an Electric Pulp Tester

16. The leukemic cells of more than 95% of patients having chronic myelogenous leukemia (CML) have a (an):
A. Missing chromosome
B. Extra chromosome
C. Philadelphia chromosome
D. New York chromosome

17. Which of the following is most often caused by retained foreign material (i.e., bone fragment etc.)?
A. Pyogenic granuloma
B. Pregnancy tumor
C. Epulis ganulomatosum
D. Fibroma

18. Which cyst listed below is extraosseous soft tissue cyst?
A. Median alveolar cyst
B. Globulomaxillary cyst
C. Nasiolabial cyst
D. Nasopalatine cyst

19. All of the statements concerning cherubism are true except:
A. It is an autosomal dominant inherited disease
B. The expansion of the jaw gives the children a very rounded face reminding one of cherubs in paintings
C. Histologically, the lesions bear a close resemblance to those seen in central giant cell granulomas
D. The treatment is radiation therapy

20. An enamel defect resulting from the incomplete formation of the enamel matrix is called:
A. Enamel pearls
B. Hypercementosis
C. Enamel hypoplasia
D. Dentinal dysplasia

21. The permanent mandibular lateral incisor typically erupts around what age?
A. 5 years old
B. 7 years old
C. 10 years old
D. 12 years old

22. The abnormal or pathological wearing away of tooth substance is referred to as:
A. Erosion
B. Attrition
C. Abrasion
D. Ablation

23. Which type of amelogenesis imperfecta is characterised by having enamel so soft that it can be removed during a prophylaxis?

A. Hypoplastic type
B. Hypocalcified type
C. Hypomaturation type
D. All of the above

24. Which of the following are characteristics of dentin dysplasia:

A. Normal enamel
B. Atypical dentin and Pulpal obliteration
C. Defective root formation
D. A tendency towards multiple periapical radiolucencies and early exfoliation of teeth
E. All of the above

25. All of the following can cause intrinsic staining of teeth except:

A. Dentinogenesis imperfecta
B. Erythroblastosis fetalis
C. Porphyria
D. Fluorosis
E. Diabetes mellitus
F. Pulpal injury
G. Internal resorption
H. Tetrcayclines

26. All of the following statements concerning benign mucous membrane pemphigoid are true except:

A. It is chronic, self-limiting, mucocutaneous disease
B. It is usually limited to the oral and ocular mucous membranes
C. It usually affects women under the age of 20
D. It is more common in the oral cavity than pemphigus, but is associated with much less morbidity and mortality

27. Mucoceles most frequently occur on the:

A. Upper lip
B. Palate
C. Lower lip
D. Gingiva

28. Which of the following infections is the one most likely to result in a chronic suppurative lesion about the jaws?

A. Actinomycosis
B. Blastomycosis
C. Histoplasmosis
D. Botryomycosis

29. The most common tumor of major and minor salivary glands is:

A. Basal cell adenoma
B. Sebaceous adenoma
C. Pleomorphic adenoma
D. Intraductal papilloma

30. The symptoms of hypothyroidism include all of the following except:

A. Feeling run down
B. Depression
C. Increased weight
D. Increased perspiration
E. Dryness and brittleness of hair
F. Dry and itchy skin
G. Constipation
H. Muscle cramps

31. Which of the following soft tissue tumors is mostly likely to be found on the tongue?

A. Traumatic neuroma
B. Neurilemmoma (Schwannoma)
C. Neurofibroma
D. None of the above

32. Which of the following are oral manifestations of patients with cerebral palsy?

A. They have a higher incidence of periodontal disease, caries, bruxism and malocclusion
B. They are prone to gingival hyperplasia if dilantin is used to control seizures
C. They are more susceptible to trauma, particularly to the maxillary anterior teeth
D. All of the above

33. A chronic condition characterized by extreme muscle weakness is called:

A. Myasthenia gravis
B. Myelofibrosis
C. Multiple sclerosis
D. Graves disease

34. Of the following types of the squamous cell carcinomas, which is the least common?

A. Squamous cell carcinoma of the palate
B. Squamous cell carcinoma of the nasopharynx
C. Squamous cell carcinoma of the oropharynx
D. Squamous cell carcinoma of the maxillary sinus

35. The most common site for necrotizing sialometaplasia is:

A. The soft plate
B. The buccal mucosa
C. The hard palate
D. The tongue

36. The peripheral giant cell granuloma always occurs on:

A. The buccal mucosa
B. The gingiva or the alveolar process
C. The lower lip
D. The palate

37. All of the following statements are true concerning Peutz-Jeghers syndrome except:

A. It is an inherited disorder, transmitted as an autosomal dominant trait
B. It is also called Hereditary lntestinal Polyposis Syndrome
C. Multiple intestinal polyps are usually distributed through the entire intestine, especially in the jejunum.
D. Melanin pigmentation of the lip and oral mucosa is usually present a birth.
E. The tongue almost invariably shows this melanin pigmentation
F. When this syndrome is suspected on the basis of oral pigmentations, other conditions to be considered in the

differential diagnosis are Addison's disease and Albright's syndrome

38. Which of the following is a characteristic of malignancy?

A. Dysplasia
B. Anaplasia
C. Metaplasia
D. All of the above

39. Primary herpes is most common in:

A. Middle age adults
B. Elderly people
C. Children and young adults
D. Infants

40. The most common viral disease of salivary gland is :

A. Sialolithiasis
B. Mumps
C. Measles
D. Candidiasis

41. A five year-old lacks sweat and sebaceous gland. He has fine, sparse hair and exhibits heat intolerance. His radiographs do not reveal tooth buds of either the primary or permanent dentition. These findings are all consistent with:

A. Pierre Robin syndrome
B. Ectodermal dysplasia
C. Cleidocranial dysostosis
D. Cherubism

42. Which of the following are symptoms of acute fluoride poisoning?

A. Nausea and abdominal pain
B. Excessive salivation
C. Vomiting & Diarrhea
D. Convulsions
E. Hypotension
F. All of the above

43. All of the following statements concerning the peripheral ossifying fibroma are true except:

A. It is most common in elderly people .
B. It usually presents as a well-demarcated focal mass of hyperplastic tissue on the gingiva with sessile or pedunculated base.
C. It is usually the same color as normal mucosa or slightly reddened.
D. It may demonstrate bone radiographically and often demonstrates bone formation histologically

44. The oral traumatic neuroma usually appears as a small nodule or swelling of the mucosa typically:

A. Near the mental foramen
B. On the alveolar ridge in edentulous areas
C. On the lips
D. On the tongue
E. All of the above

45. Which form of ameloblastoma is the more aggressive one and requires more extensive treatment?

A. Solid (multicystic)
B. Unicystic
C. Extraosseous
D. All of the above

46. Which of the following is defined as a persistent velvety red patch that cannot be characterized clinically as any other condition?

A. Leukoedema
B. Psoriasis
C. Erythroplakia
D. White sponge nevus

47. Median rhomboid glossitis frequently affects:

A. Toddlers
B. Infants
C. Middle-aged adults
D. Teenagers

48. Which malignant salivary gland tumor listed below most often occurs in the minor salivary gland of the palate?

A. Adenoid cystic carcinoma
B. Mucoepidermoid carcinoma
C. Pleomorphic adenoma
D. None of the above

49. A persons with mucormycosis generally is treated with:

A. Penicillin
B. Erythromycin
C. Amphotericin B
D. Clindamycin

50. All of the following statements concerning syphilis are true excepts:

A. It is a sexually transmitted disease caused by a bacterium called Treponema palidum (a spirochete).
B. It occurs in 3 stage, viz. primary, secondary and tertiary.
C. First symptom of primary syphilis is chancre.
D. It is usually treated with tetracycline injections.

51. "Burning tongue syndrome" typically affects:

A. Children
B. Teenagers
C. Middle-aged females
D. Middle-aged males

52. All of the following statements concerning the central ossifying fibroma of bone are true except:

A. It is a slow-growing, painless, asymptomatic neoplasm which may occur in either jaw
B. It may occur at any age, but it is far more common in elderly people
C. The displacement of teeth may be an early clinical feature
D. Because of this slow growth, the cortical plates of bone and overlying mucosa and skin are almost always invariably intact.

53. A malignant tumor developing from bone marrow, usually in long bones or the pelvis of adolescent boys is called

A. Myeloma
B. Ewing's sarcoma

C. Osteogenic sarcoma
D. Multiple myeloma

54. A severe bullous form of erythema multiforme is known as:
A. Plummer- Vinson syndrome
B. Peutz- Jeghers syndrome
C. Gardener's syndrome
D. Stevens- Johnson syndrome

55. Which type of acquired nevi listed below is the most common variety seen in the oral cavity?
A. Intradermal Nevus
B. Compound nevus
C. Junctional nevus
D. Blue nevus
E. Intramucosal nevus

56. An acute condition characterized by pronounced leukopenia with a severe reduction in the number of polymorphonuclear leukocytes is called:
A. Infectious mononucleosis
B. Agranulocytosis
C. Sickle-cell anemia
D. Porphyria

57. Which virus listed below can cause herpes zoster lesions along sensory nerve roots in later life?
A. Pox virus
B. Epstein - Barr virus
C. Varicella virus
D. Mumps virus

58. The treatment of choice for Sjogren syndrome is:
A. Radiation
B. Surgical excision
C. Chemotherapy
D. None of the above

59. All of the following are oral or para-oral presentations of herpes simplex except:
A. Acute herpetic gingivostomatitis

B. Herpes digitalis
C. Recurrent herpetic stomatitis
D. Herpes labialis

60. Cementomas (periapical cemental dyplasia) occur most frequently in the:
A. Mandible
B. Maxilla
C. Zygoma
D. Clavicle

61. Which of the following odontogenic tumors have a mixed origin (ectodermal- mesodermal) ?
A. Ameloblastic fibroma
B. Ameloblastic fibro-odontoma
C. Ameloblastic odontoma
D. All of the above

62. Which neoplasm listed below has strong evidence of a viral etiology?
A. Ewing's sarcoma
B. Burkitt's lymphoma
C. Liposarcoma
D. Osteoid osteoma

63. The central giant cell granuloma occurs predominantly in:
A. Infants
B. Children or young adults
C. Middle aged adults
D. Elderly people

64. Oral lesions are most likely to be observed in:
A. Myelogenous leukemia
B. Lymphocytic leukemia
C. Monocytic leukemia
D. Myelo-monocytic leukemia

65. An inability to absorb adequate amounts of vitamin B_{12} from the digestive tract may result in:
A. Thalassemia
B. Pernicious anemia

C. Aplastic anemia
D. None of the above

66. There is increasing evidence that Mikukicz's disease is closely related to:
A. Pierre-Robin syndrome
B. Sjogren's syndrome
C. Goltz-Gorlin syndrome
D. Apert syndrome

67. Recurrent aphthous ulcers:
A. Are caused by the Epstein-Barr virus
B. Are caused by the Herpes Simplex virus
C. Appear to be associated with stress
D. Are caused by a Poxvirus

68. Occlusal radiographs are useful in locating:
A. The hyoid bone
B. The mental foramen
C. Sialoliths in Wharton's duct
D. Sialoliths in Stensen's duct

69. A chronic skin disease that is characterized by the formation of vesicles and bullae is called:
A. Lichen planus
B. Candidiasis
C. White sponge nevus
D. Pemphigus

70. Hairy tongue is a condition characterized by hypertrophy of the:
A. Filiform papillae
B. Fungiform papillae
C. Circumvallate papillae
D. Foliate papillae

71. The characteristic lesion of erythema multiforme is:
A. Melanin pigmentation
B. A chancre
C. The "bull's-eye- shaped" lesion
D. A blister

72. A poorly differentiated squamous carcinoma involving lymphoid tissues in the region of the tonsils and nasopharynx is called:

A. A lipoma
B. A lymphoepithelioma
C. A lymphoma
D. A nasopharyngioma

73. The most common form of fibrous dysplasia is:

A. Monostotic
B. Polyostotic
C. Polyostotic with endocrine involvement (Albright's syndrome)
D. All of the above.

74. Which of the following is also known as Rendu-Osler-Weber disease?

A. Hereditary hemorrhagic telangiectasia
B. Encephalotrigeminal angiomatosis
C. Juvenile nasopharyngeal angiofibroma
D. Hereditary intestinal polyposis

75. All of the following statements are true concerning the aneurysmal bone cyst except:

A. It is an uncommon expansile osteolytic lesion of bone consisting of a proliferation of vascular tissue that forms a lining around blood filled cystic lesions
B. Most aneurysmal bone cysts occur in patients under 20 years of age, and it is uncommon after the age of 30
C. It commonly involves the jaws
D. The lesions are usually tender or painful particularly upon motion of the bone affected
E. Upon entering the lesion surgically, excessive bleeding is encountered

76. The most common form of malignant melanoma is

A. Superficial spreading
B. Nodular
C. Acrolentiginous
D. Lentigo maligna

77. Which type of a cancer listed below occurs most frequently in the oral cavity?

A. Basal cell carcinoma
B. Squamous cell carcinoma
C. Angiosarcoma
D. Pindborg tumor

78. The etiology of leukemia is:

A. Viral
B. Bacterial
C. Fungal
D. Unknown

79. An unusual phenomenon, with arises as a result of damage to the auriculotemporal nerve and subsequent reinnervation of the sweat glands by parasympathetic salivary fibers is called:

A. Postherpetic neuralgia
B. Orolingual paresthesia
C. Frey's syndrome
D. Glossopharyngeal neuralgia

80. The multiple endocrine neoplasia syndromes are a group of syndromes characterized by:

A. Tumors of the CNS
B. Tumors of the skin
C. Tumors of the various endocrine glands
D. Tumors of the salivary glands

81. A condition characterized by hemorrhages in the skin and mucous membranes that results in the appearance of purplish spots or patches is called:

A. Addison's disease
B. Purpura
C. Aplastic anemia
D. Hemophilia

82. Lateral clefting of the lip results from the failure of:

A. The maxillary processes to merge
B. The palatine processes to merge
C. The maxillary and frontonasal processes to merge
D. None of the above

83. A periapical abscess usually arises as a result of:
A. Orthodontics
B. Trauma
C. Infection of the pulp of a tooth
D. Periodontal disease

84. All of the following statements concerning eosinophilic granuloma are true except:
A. It tends to start between the age of 50 and 70
B. It affects males more than females
C. It usually affects the bones but also affects the lungs
D. Clinically, the lesions may present no physical signs or symptoms.

85. Which of the following terms refers to a small section of tissue that is removed for examination?
A. Excisional biopsy
B. Incisional biopsy
C. FNAC
D. Neither of the above

86. All of the following statements concerning craniofacial fibrous dysplasia are true except:
A. This condition frequently causes expansion and deformity of the jaw bones, as well as displacement of the teeth.
B. There is a characteristic thickening at the base of the skull, which can be seen radiographically.
C. Radiographically, the lesion is usually radiopaque, not well-circumscribed, and may have a "ground-glass" appearance.
D. The treatment of choice is radiation therapy
E. It is also referred to as "monostotic" fibrous dysplasia of the jaw

87. The most common site for carcinoma of the tongue is the:
A. Dorsum
B. Tip
C. Lateral border
D. Sulcus terminalis

88. A form of leukemia in which the abnormal cells are thought to be the precursors of lymphoblasts, myeloblasts, monoblasts is called:

A. Aleukemic leukemia
B. Subleukemic leukemia
C. Stem cell leukemia
D. None of the above

89. Excessive formation of cementum on the surface of the root is referred to as:

A. Cemental pearls
B. Hypercementosis
C. Secondary cementum
D. Condensing osteitis

90. The nevoid basal cell carcinoma syndrome may present which of the following abnormalities?

A. Cutaneous anomalies
B. Dental and osseous anomalies
C. Ophthalmologic abnormalities
D. Neurologic anomalies
E. Sexual abnormalities
F. All of the above

91. All of the statements concerning chronic leukemia are true except:

A. It has an abrupt onset
B. The skin is frequently involved in chronic leukemia and may manifest as petechiae or ecchymoses.
C. Massive splenomegaly is characteristic of chronic myelogenous leukemia.
D. Lymph node enlargement is the main pathologic finding in chronic lymphocytic leukemia

92. The term iatrogenic refers to:

A. A disease or condition of unknown cause or origin
B. A condition caused by medical personnel or procedures
C. A tissue or an organ transferred into a new position within the body of the same individual
D. Any of the above

93. All of the following statements concerning Addison's disease are true except:

A. It is a rare endocrine disorder which occurs when the adrenal glands do not produce enough cortisol.
B. It is sometimes called chronic adrenal insufficiency or hypocorticolism.
C. It most commonly affects teenagers
D. It afflicts men and women equally
E. It is characterized by weight loss, muscles weakness, low blood pressure, and darkening of the skin in both exposed and unexposed parts of the body.

94. After the initial primary attack during the early childhood period, the herpes simplex virus remains inactive most commonly in the

A. Geniculate ganglion
B. Ciliary ganglion
C. Trigeminal ganglion
D. Pterygopalatine ganglion

95. All of the following statements concerning developmental salivary gland defects are true except:

A. They are very common
B. They are asymptomatic
C. They are next to impossible to palpate manually
D. They are discovered only during radiographic examination of the area

96. All of the following statements concerning malignant melanoma are true except:

A. It is relatively benign form of skin cancer
B. Currently about 1 in 100 persons in the United States can except to develop this cancer in a lifetime.
C. Without treatment, it has the tendency to become widely metastatic and result in the demise of the patient
D. There are four general clinical types of melanoma i.e. superficial spreading, nodular acrolentiginous and lentigo maligna

97. Kaposi's sarcoma is an oral manifestation of:

A. Diabetes
B. Hypothyroidism
C. AIDS
D. Lichen planus

98. All of the following statements concerning amelogenesis imperfecta are true except:

A. It is an inherited condition which is transmitted as a dominant trait
B. It only effects the permanent teeth
C. It causes the enamel of the teeth to be soft and thin
D. The teeth appear yellow, because the dentin is visible through the thin enamel
E. The teeth are easily damaged and susceptible to decay

99. An incisional biopsy is indicated for which of the following lesions?

A. A 5 cm papillary fibroma of the gingiva
B. A 2 cm exostosis of the hard palate.
C. A 2 cm area of Fordyce's disease of the cheek
D. A 3 cm hemangioma of the tongue
E. A 3 cm area of leukoplakia of the soft palate

100. All of the following metabolic conditions are associated with chronic salivary gland enlargement except:

A. Diabetes mellitus
B. Chronic alcoholism
C. Malnutrition (including anorexia and bulimia)
D. Hypothyroidism

101. Which of the following is one of the most important substances that influences the rate of healing of wounds in the oral cavity?

A. Fat
B. Protein
C. Iron
D. Calcium

102. Actinic cheilitis is caused by:

A. A virus
B. Stress
C. Chronic and excessive exposure to the ultraviolet radiation in sunlight
D. Certain medications

103. Osteogenesis imperfecta is caused by a genetic defect that affects the body's production of:

A. Viamin K
B. Collagen
C. Reticulin
D. Elastin

104. All of the following statements concerning condensing osteitis are true except:

A. It most often occurs in young patients
B. The mandibular second molar is the tooth most commonly involved
C. It is most often seen associated with a long -standing periapical infection
D. There may be no signs or symptoms of the disease other than mild pain associated with an infected pulp.

105. Condylar hyperplasia is:

A. A common, bilateral enlargement of the condyle
B. A rare, bilateral enlargement of the condyle
C. A common, unilateral enlargement of the condyle
D. A rare, unilateral enlargement of the condyle

106. All of the following are characterized by granulomatous inflammation except:

A. Sarcoidosis
B. Tuberculosis
C. Pneumonia
D. Histoplasmosis
E. Tertiary syphilis

107. All of the following statements concerning an osteosarcoma are true except:

A. It is a malignant bone tumor composed of anaplastic tissue derived from mesenchyme.

B. Its peak incidence is after epiphyseal fusion, particularly the years between 50 and 60.

C. This tumor seems to arise in the long bones, which show the greatest longitudinal growth.

D. Joint involvement is rare

108. A severe hemolytic disease of the fetus / newborn caused by the production of maternal antibodies for fetal red blood cells is called:

A. Sickle- cell anemia

B. Erythroblastosis fetalis

C. Erythrocyanosis

D. Aplastic anemia

109. The fusion of the alveolar bone to a tooth is known as:

A. Hypercementosis

B. Gomphosis

C. Ankylosis

D. Gemination

110. In an OPG of a 14-year-old patient, a large radiolucent area on the left side of the mandible apical to the premolars and first molar is seen. No clinical symptoms are present. Teeth are not carious and respond normally to vitality tests. Medical history is unremarkable. Upon opening in to the area, no fluid or tissue is evident. What is the most probable diagnosis?

A. Dentigerous cyst

B. Traumatic bone cyst

C. Primordial cyst

D. Residual cyst

111. All of the following statements concerning polycythemia vera are true except:

A. It is characterized by excessive erythrocyte production

B. It usually occurs within the age range of 10-35, with 20 being the mean age of onset

C. Polycythemia vera is considered to be one of the chronic myeloproliferative disorders
D. Clinical features include headaches, weakness, weight loss, and pruritus
E. Hemorrhage and thrombosis may be evident at any time

112. A patient is observed to have a drooping mouth on one side and a watering eye. She complains of having a loss of taste sensation on the anterior portion of her tongue. This patient is most likely suffering from:
A. Cerebral palsy
B. Bell's palsy
C. Tic douloureux
D. Multiple sclerosis

113. When using the TNM method in assessing the prognosis and therapy of malignant neoplasms, the N represents:
A. The presence of Nikolsky's sign
B. The presence of nodules
C. The presence of regional lymph node involvement
D. The presence of erythroplakia.

114. All of the following statements concerning Plummer-Vinson syndrome are true except:
A. It is a rare disorder associated with severe and chronic iron-deficiency anemia
B. It occurs chiefly in adolescent teenagers
C. Systemic symptoms include weakness, pallor, difficulty in swallowing and difficulty in breathing
D. Oral symptoms include angular stomatitis and a smooth, red painful tongue with atrophy of the papillae

115. All of the following statements concerning acute leukemia are true except:
A. It has an insidious onset
B. Acute myelogenous leukemia is more common in adults
C. Acute Lymphocytic Leukemia is largely confined to children.
D. Symptoms include severe anemia, hemorrhages, and slight enlargement of the lymph nodes or the spleen

116. All of the following are histological characteristics of malignancy except:
A. Abnormal mitosis
B. Metaplasia
C. Pleomorphism
D. Hyperchromatism
E. Anaplasia
F. Increased nuclear-cytoplasmic ratio

117. The leukemic cells of more than 95% of patients having chronic myelogenous leukemia (CML) have a (an):
A. Missing chromosome
B. Extra chromosome
C. Philadelphia chromosome
D. New York chromosome

118. Benign migratory glossitis is also known as:
A. Fissured tongue
B. Macroglossia
C. Geographic tongue
D. Hairy tongue

119. The general characteristics listed below describe malignant neoplasm except ?
A. Invasion
B. Movable
C. Rapid growth
D. Metastasis
E. Not well- differentiated (or anaplastic)

120. All of the following cysts are congenital except:
A. Thyroglossal duct cyst
B. Branchiogenic cyst
C. Globulomaxillary cyst
D. Dermoid cyst

121. All of the following are dental manifestations of hypoparathyroidism except:
A. Delayed eruption of teeth
B. Small tooth crowns with short crown/root ratio

C. Blunted root apices
D. Enamel hypoplasia

122. All of the following statements concerning metastatic tumors of the jaws are true except:
A. They may be completely asymptomatic
B. The patient is usually aware of slight discomfort or pain
C. The maxilla is affected far more frequently than the mandible
D. The molar region is predominantly involved

123. All of the following diseases have traditionally been grouped under the generic term Histiocytosis X except:
A. Eosinophilic granuloma
B. Tay-Sachs disease
C. Hand Schuller-Christian disease
D. Letterer- Siwe disease

124. All of the following statements concerning verrucous carcinoma are true except:
A. It is rare form of squamous cell carcinoma that occurs in either the oral or laryngeal cavity
B. There is a characteristic whitish, cauliflower, or coral appearance to the mass
C. Typically, the lesion develops on the vocal cords of an elderly male who has been a heavy cigarette smoker
D. It is known for its slow growth pattern and well-developed hyperkeratotic epithelial boundaries
E. It usually shows rapid metastasis

125. A malignancy of plasma cells is called:
A. Histoplasmosis
B. Multiple myeloma
C. Osteomalacia
D. Amyloidosis

126. Oncocytomas are true tumors that may occur:
A. In the kidney
B. In the salivary glands
C. In endocrine gland
D. All of the above

127. Which of the following are thought to be predisposing factors to the development of angular cheilitis (perleche):
A. Intraoral infection by Candida albicans
B. Loss of intermaxillary distance (decreased vertical dimension)
C. Trauma to the commissure induced by prolonged dental treatment
D. Vitamin deficiencies (particularly riboflavin or thiamine)
E. All of the above

128. A condition that mimics leukoplakia in that it seems to be a white patch is called
A. Leukemia
B. Leukemoid
C. Leukoedema
D. Leukochloroma

129. The inflammation or infection of the bone marrow and adjacent bone is called
A. Osteopetrosis
B. Osteoporosis
C. Osteomyelitis
D. Osteonecrosis

130. Which type of hepatitis is also know as "Serum Hepatitis"?
A. Hepatitis A
B. Hepatitis B
C. Hepatitis AB
D. Hepatitis C

131. The cause of infectious mononucleosis is:
A. The pox virus
B. The Epstein- Barr virus
C. The rubella virus
D. The paramyxovirus

132. An uncommon hereditary disorder characterized principally by the overgrowth and denseness of bones is called:
A. Osteopetrosis
B. Osteogenesis imperfecta

C. Achondroplasia
D. Fibrous dysplasia

133. In the African form of Burkitt's lymphoma:
A. The patients are generally older than in the non- African form
B. The patients are generally younger than in the non-African form
C. There is no gender predilection
D. It presents most often as an abdominal mass

134. Mandibular tori most often appear:
A. In the retromolar pad region
B. On the lingual surface of the mandible, most often in the premolar region
C. On the lingual surface of the mandible, inferior to the mylohyoid ridge
D. Along the midline of the hard palate

135. Follicular and dentigerous cysts that contain keratinizing material are known as:
A. Residual cysts
B. Traumatic bone cysts
C. Keratocysts
D. Granulomas

136. In most cases, what is the proper treatment for an eruption cyst?
A. Incise and drain
B. Prescribe antibiotics
C. No treatment is necessary
D. Extract the tooth associated with the eruption cyst

137. Which of the following may occur at any age and presents as a single or multiple small, flat brown asymptomatic lesions occurring mostly on the lower lip?
A. Blue nevus
B. Compound nevus
C. Focal melanosis
D. Lipoma

138. The most common location for an intraoral congenital nevi (birthmark) is the

A. Buccal mucosa
B. Tongue
C. Hard palate
D. Alveolar mucosa

139. All of the following statements concerning acromegaly are true except:

A. It is a hormonal disorder that results when the pituitary gland produces excess ACTH.
B. It most commonly affects middle-aged adults and can result in serious illness and premature death.
C. Soft tissue swelling of the hands and feet is often an early feature, with patients noticing a change in ring or shoe size.
D. Gradually, body changes alter the patient's facial features (i.e., the brow and lower jaw protrude, the nasal bone enlarges ,and spacing of the teeth increases)

140. The erythrocyte sedimentation rate (ESR) is a nonspecific test that monitors

A. Bleeding rate
B. The progression of disease
C. Prothrombin time
D. Platelet function

141. The most common primary malignant tumor of bone is:

A. An osteosarcoma
B. A chondrosarcoma
C. Ewing's sarcoma
D. A myeloma

142. Which of the following types of skin cancer is considered to be the most severe?

A. Basal cell carcinoma
B. Squamous cell carcinoma
C. Malignant melanoma
D. Fibroma

143. All of the following cysts occur with in bone except:
A. The nasopalatine cyst
B. The median palatal cyst
C. The nasiolabial cyst
D. The globulomaxillary cyst

144. All of the following are characteristics of Gardner's syndrome except:
A. This syndrome is inherited in a dominant manner
B. Thousands of polyps develop in the colon, as well as the stomach and duodenum
C. This syndrome is also associated with bony tumors in the jaw and skull
D. The polyps rarely undergo malignant transformation

145. Xerostomia is caused by:
A. Sialadenitis
B. Sjogren's syndrome
C. Medications
D. Cancer therapy
E. Nerve damage
F. Conditions such as Alzheimer's disease or stroke, bone marrow transplants, endocrine disorders, stress, anxiety, depression and nutritional deficiencies
G. All of the above

146. An increased serum alkaline phosphatase level is clinically significant and aids in the diagnosis of
A. Hyperparathyroidism
B. Paget's disease of bone
C. Myasthenia gravis
D. Prostate cancer

147. Hypophosphatasia is one of several disorders that resembles:
A. Acromegaly
B. Paget' disease
C. Osteogenesis imperfecta
D. Ewing's sarcoma

148. Ludwig's angina refers to cellulitis of the floor of the mouth, in which the infection spreads to the:

A. Submental space
B. Sublingual space
C. Submandibular space
D. All of the above

149. All of the following statements concerning white sponge nevus are true except:

A. It is an autosomal dominant condition
B. It is also called familial white folded dysplasia
C. It is characterized by soft, white, or opalescent, thickened and corrugated folds of mucous membrane
D. The treatment for white sponge nevus is surgical excision and radiation

150. The most common form of recurrent aphthous stomatitis is:

A. Recurrent aphthous minor
B. Recurrent aphthous major
C. Recurrent herpetiform
D. Herpetic lesions

151. What is the most probable diagnosis for a lesion that presents as a translucent, bluish, well- rounded, smooth surfaced and protrudes from one side of the floor of the mouth?

A. A mucocele
B. Squamous cell carcinoma
C. A ranula
D. A lymphangioma

152. Which of the of the following cysts is most commonly found in relation to a developing third molar?

A. Lateral periodontal cysts
B. Dentigerous cyst
C. Fissural cyst
D. Primordial cyst
E. Traumatic cysts
F. Residual cyst
G. Gingival cyst

153. A developmental abnormality characterized by the total absence of teeth is called:

A. Hypodontia
B. Anodontia
C. Diphyodontia
D. Hypsodontia

154. Which of the following bone lesions is most likely to be fatal?

A. Osteochondroma
B. Paget's disease
C. Giant cell tumor
D. Multiple myeloma
E. Odontogenic myxoma

155. Which form of hepatitis is caused by an RNA enterovirus and is usually transmitted by the fecal - oral route?

A. Hepatitis A
B. Hepatitis B
C. Hepatitis C
D. Hepatitis E

156. The etiology of verruca vulgaris is:

A. Fungal
B. Bacterial
C. Viral
D. Parasitic

157. All of the following tests can be used to diagnose herpetic lesions except

A. The Tzanck smear
B. Fluorescent staining
C. An arthrogram
D. Isolation in tissue culture
E. Antibody titers
F. Biopsy

158. Which term listed below is a development defect characterized by an overgrowth of tissue not normal to the organ in which it arises?

A. Teratoma
B. Choristoma

C. Hamartoma
D. Lipoma

159. An acute infectious disease caused by a group a coxsackie virus is called:
A. Herpes zoster
B. Chickenpox
C. Herpangina
D. Herpes labialis

160. All of the following are clinical features of benign salivary gland tumors except:
A. Mucosa is normal
B. Painless
C. Nodular
D. Movable
E. Fixed
F. Firm
G. Slow-growing

161. All of the followings statements concerning oral candidiasis are true except:
A. It is also called "thrush"
B. It is a bacterial infection of the mouth
C. It is most often caused by Candida albicans
D. The most common symptoms of oral candidiasis are discomfort and burning of the mouth and throat and an altered taste
E. Antibiotics prescribed for a dental infection may cause oral candidiasis

162. Warthin's tumor is almost exclusively seen in the:
A. Submandibular gland
B. Sublingual gland
C. Parotid gland
D. Minor salivary glands

163. All of the following statements concerning osteomalacia are true except:
A. Osteomalacia means hardening of the bones
B. The signs and symptoms include pain in the arm, legs, spine, and pelvis

C. It is the adult form of Rickets
D. One of the most common causes is a problem of fat malabsorption called steatorrhea.

164. The symptoms of hyperthyroidism include all of the following except:
A. Nervousness
B. Irritability
C. Increased perspiration
D. Constipation
E. Fine brittle hair
F. Muscular weakness
G. Weight loss despite a good appetite

165. All of the following cysts are developmental (or fissural except:
A. Nasopalatine cyst
B. Nasolabial cyst
C. Globulomaxillary cyst
D. Branchiogenic cyst
E. Median palatal cyst
F. Median alveolar cyst

166. Inflammatory papillary hyperplasia is found on the:
A. Soft palate
B. Buccal mucosa
C. Hard palate
D. Tongue

167. All of the following are clinical features of malignant salivary gland tumors except:
A. Mucosa is ulcerated
B. Painless
C. Nodular
D. Firm
E. Fixed
F. Rapid growth

168. A white patch on the oral mucosa that cannot be rubbed off and cannot be assigned to any other disease is most probably:

A. Candidiasis
B. Lichen planus
C. Leukoplakia
D. Erythroplakia

169. Acinic cell carcinoma is a malignant salivary gland tumor that is most likely to be associated with the:

A. Submandibular gland
B. Parotid gland
C. Sublingual gland
D. Minor gland of the palate

170. The term used to describe permanent incisors which may be characteristic of congenital syphilis is:

A. Blandi's incisors
B. Turner's incisors
C. Franklin's incisors
D. Hutchinson's incisors

Answer Key to MCQs in Oral Pathology

1	C	2	A	3	C	4	C
5	D	6	B	7	B	8	A
9	B	10	D	11	C	12	B
13	B	14	A	15	C	16	C
17	C	18	C	19	D	20	C
21	B	22	C	23	B	24	E
25	E	26	C	27	C	28	A
29	C	30	D	31	B	32	D
33	A	34	B	35	C	36	B
37	E	38	D	39	C	40	B
41	B	42	F	43	A	44	B
45	A	46	C	47	C	48	A
49	C	50	D	51	C	52	B
53	B	54	D	55	E	56	B

57	C	58	D	59	B	60	A
61	D	62	B	63	B	64	C
65	B	66	B	67	C	68	C
69	D	70	A	71	C	72	B
73	A	74	A	75	C	76	A
77	B	78	D	79	C	80	C
81	B	82	C	83	C	84	A
85	B	86	D	87	C	88	C
89	B	90	F	91	A	92	B
93	C	94	C	95	A	96	A
97	C	98	B	99	E	100	D
101	B	102	C	103	B	104	B
105	D	106	C	107	B	108	B
109	C	110	B	111	B	112	B
113	C	114	B	115	A	116	B
117	C	118	C	119	B	120	C
121	B	122	C	123	B	124	E
125	B	126	D	127	E	128	C
129	C	130	B	131	B	132	A
133	B	134	B	135	C	136	C
137	C	138	C	139	A	140	B
141	A	142	C	143	C	144	D
145	G	146	B	147	C	148	D
149	D	150	A	151	C	152	B
153	B	154	D	155	A	156	C
157	C	158	B	159	C	160	E
161	B	162	C	163	A	164	D
165	D	166	C	167	B	168	C
169	B	170	D				

19

MCQs in General Medicine

Part I

1. Bilateral lower motor neurone facial palsy can be caused by:
A. Leprosy
B. Mumps
C. Sarcoidosis
D. Tabes dorsalis

2. During CPR, the effectiveness of cardiac massage is indicated by:
A. Increase in pulse rate more than 60 per minute
B. Increase in pulsation in great veins
C. Disappearance of cyanosis
D. Pulsations appear and the constriction of pupil starts

3. Parkinsonism can be indicated which of the following:
A. Lead pipe rigidity
B. Positive Romberg's sign
C. Loss of position sense
D. Loss of fine touch

4. A viral infection which responds to antibiotics is:
A. Chickenpox
B. Lymphogranuloma venerum
C. Measles
D. Mumps

5. Which of the following is not seen in hyperaldosteronism:
   A. ↑ Calcium
   B. Hypertension
   C. Hypokalemia
   D. Polyuria

6. Which of the following is not a sex-linked disease:
   A. Duchenne type myopathy
   B. G-6-P D deficiency
   C. Galactosemia
   D. Hemophilia

7. All of the following can be seen in zinc deficiency except:
   A. Acrodermatitis
   B. Decreased wound healing
   C. Goitre
   D. Hypogonadism

8. Hyperkalemia is treated with:
   A. Glucagon
   B. Insulin
   C. Corticosteroids
   D. Ringer lactate

9. In resistant congestive heart failure, diuretic of choice is:
   A. Triamterene
   B. Spironolactone
   C. Furosemide
   D. Acetazolamide

10. Which of the following is true about HLA:
   A. It can be changed with immunosuppresives
   B. It is determined on neutrophils
   C. It is not useful for determining paternity
   D. It is useful to determine paternity

11. Treatment of ventricular fibrillation is:
   A. Immediate electrical cardio-version
   B. Intravenous digoxin
   C. Intravenous propranolol
   D. Intravenous soda bicarbonate

12. Left ventricular failure is indicated, if pulmonary artery wedge pressure exceeds:

A. 5 mm Hg
B. 10 mm Hg
C. 15 mm Hg
D. 20 mm Hg

13. Following is the most important factor in the management of shock:

A. Blood pressure
B. Cardiac output
C. CVP to 8 cm of water
D. Deficiency of effective circulating blood volume

14. SABE does not occur in:

A. ASD
B. Small VSD
C. Fallot's Tetralogy
D. Mitral valve prolapse.

15. Gram negative septic shock is most commonly due to infection of:

A. Biliary tract
B. Genitourinary tract
C. GIT
D. Respiratory tract

16. Which statement is true for staphylococcal pneumonia:

A. Common after viral infection
B. Interstitial long tissue involved
C. Multiple lung abscesses common
D. Resolution occurs without scar
E. Upper posterior lobe most often involved

17. Congenitally passed immunity is not observed with:

A. Chickenpox
B. Mumps
C. Poliomyelitis
D. Rubella
E. Whooping cough

18. Ideal treatment for thalassemia is:
A. Packed cells
B. Platelets
C. Washed cells
D. Whole blood

19. Chvostek' and Trousseau's signs positive and hyperreflexia denote the deficiency of:
A. Calcium
B. Magnesium
C. Potassium
D. Sodium

20. The following disease is most likely to cause syncope and angina in the same patient:
A. Ischemic Heart Disease
B. Aortic stenosis
C. Mitral valve prolapse
D. Vertebro-basilar artery insufficiency

21. K^+ depletion occurs is:
A. Addison's disease
B. Diarrhoea
C. Pheochromocytoma
D. Renal failure

22. Of the HLA, most significant is:
A. HLA—A
B. HLA—B
C. HLA—C
D. HLA—D

23. Hemiplegia is most often caused by thrombosis of:
A. Anterior cerebral artery
B. Basilar artery
C. Middle cerebral artery
D. Posterior cerebral artery

24. Marfan's Syndrome involves all of the following except:
A. Abnormalities of eyes
B. Long tapering fingers

C. Marked obesity
D. Dissecting aneurysm

25. Sturge-Weber syndrome is:
A. An outcome of bilateral temporal lobes ablation
B. A tumor of pituitary with gigantism
C. A sequela of head injury
D. Multiple angiomas over face, eyes and brain

26. Drug of choice in chronic myeloid leukaemia is:
A. Busulphan
B. Chlorambucil
C. Leukeran
D. Melphalan

27. The treatment of hypoxic hypoxia is:
A. Bronchodilators
B. Hyperbaric oxygen
C. Pure oxygen
D. Vasodilators

28. Most specific urinary finding in acute glomerulonephritis is:
A. Cellular (RBC's) casts
B. WBC's casts
C. Albuminuria
D. Serum creatinine

29. In thalassemia following are seen except:
A. Target cells
B. Mongoloid facies
C. ↑ Osmotic fragility
D. Microcytic hypochromic anemia

30. Which is not a feature of diabetic ketoacidosis:
A. Kussmauli's breathing
B. Ataxia
C. Tremors
D. Severe dehydration

31. HLA—DR 4 is marker of:
A. Rheumatoid arthritis
B. Sarcoidosis

C. Seronegative gouty arthritis
D. Psoriasis

32. Earliest symptom of myasthenia is:
A. Diplopia + ptosis
B. Fatigue
C. Respiratory weakness
D. Palatal palsy

33. Petecheal haemorrhages seen in the gums is due to the deficiency of:
A. Vitamin K
B. Ascorbic acid
C. Cholecalciferol
D. Nicotinic acid

34. Diabetic coma is caused by:
A. Ketosis
B. Hyperglycemia with hyper-osmolar ketosis
C. Hyperkalemia
D. Simple hyperglycemia

35. The skin pigmentation in bronze diabetes is due to:
A. Hemosiderin
B. Lipofuschin
C. Melanin
D. Ceroids

36. 'Kala Azar' is treated with compound of:
A. Gold
B. Bismuth
C. Antimony
D. Mercury

37. The following drug may lead to occurrence of Parkinsonism:
A. Bromocriptine
B. Levodopa
C. Methyl dopa
D. Carbidopa

38. Metabolic acidosis occur in:
A. Hyperaldosteronism
B. Excessive liquor ingestion

C. Milk - alkali syndrome
D. Diarrhoea

39. "Peu-de orange" may be seen in:
A. G-6-P-D deficiency
B. Alcoholism
C. Hurler's syndrome
D. Hunter's syndrome

40. "Casal's Necklace" and "Crazy pavement" is seen in"
A. Beri-Beri
B. Scabies
C. Pityriasis rosea
D. Pellagra

41. The vitamin contraindicated in therapy with levodopa is:'
A. B_2
B. Pyridoxine
C. Folic acid
D. Ascorbic acid

42. In metabolic acidosis, respiration is:
A. Deep and slow
B. Deep and sighing
C. Slow and superficial
D. Cheyne Stokes type

43. For excessive sweating, the intravenous fluid of choice is:
A. Dextrose saline
B. Ringer lactate
C. Dextran
D. Plasma

44. The worst complication of high altitude is:
A. Hypoxia
B. Pulmonary oedema
C. Polycythemia
D. Fits

45. The commonest cause of stroke in an elderly is:
A. Thrombosis
B. Embolism

C. Atrial fibrillation
D. Berry aneurysm rupture

46. Best treatment of diabetic ketoacidosis is:
A. 2 hourly insulin
B. 6 hourly insulin
C. Slow infusion with insulin
D. Large bolus of insulin subcutaneously

47. The commonest cause of pulmonary embolism:
A. Superficial cause of pulmonary embolism
B. Deep vein thrombosis
C. Pelvic vein thrombosis
D. Heart failure

48. Major criteria of rheumatic fever includes:
A. Erythema nodosum
B. Subcutaneous nodules
C. ↑ ASO titre
D. Fever

49. Sinus bradycardia is seen in:
A. Hypothyroidism
B. 1st degree block
C. Grave's disease
D. Adrenalectomy

50. 4th Heart sound is Heard in:
A. Early systole
B. Early diastole
C. Late systole
D. Late diastole

51. Enzyme raised within hours of MI & lasts 2-3 days is:
A. LDH
B. CPK
C. AST
D. ALT

52. In hypoparathyroidism:
A. Ionic Ca^{2+} levels are ↓
B. Kidney stones

C. Urinary Ca_2+ ↓
D. Total serum calcium is normal

53. All serum proteins are reduced in nephritic syndrome except:
A. Albumin
B. Transferrin
C. Ceruloplasmin
D. Fibrinogen

54. X - linked recessive disease is characterized by:
A. Vertical transmission
B. 50 % female carriers if male is affected
C. 50 % male affected if female is diseased
D. 50 % male carriers if female is diseased

55. Muscles not usually involved in polymyositis are:
A. Limb muscles
B. Ocular muscles
C. Pharyngeal muscles
D. Jaw muscles

56. Rx of choice in a case of acute MI with arrythmias is:
A. Procainamide
B. Lignocaine
C. Quinidin
D. Digoxin

57. Ectopic ACTH is most commonly produced by:
A. Lung carcinoma
B. Carcinoma breast
C. Ca prostate
D. Adrenal tumors

58. Myaesthenia gravis is associated with:
A. Hyperparathyroidism
B. Thymoma
C. Ca lung
D. Thyroid carcinoma

59. A negative Montoux test is of significance in one of the following conditions:
A. Pulmonary TB

B. Silicosis
C. Sarcoidosis .
D. Wegner's granulomatosis

60. All may be seen during fasting except:
A. Hypoglycemia
B. Hypercholesteroleamia
C. Hyperlipidemia
D. Keto acidosis

61. Rubella leads to following except:
A. PS pulmonary stenosis
B. ASD atrial septal defect
C. VSD ventricular septal defect
D. PDA patent ductus arteriosus

62. Following are the causes of microcytic hypochromic anemia except:
A. Iron deficiency
B. Thalassemia
C. Hypothyroidism
D. Sideroblastic anemia

63. Dawn phenomenon refers to:
A. Early morning hypoglycemia
B. Non-ketotic hypercalcaemia
C. After breakfast hypercalcaemia
D. Recurrent hypoglycemia

64. Exposure to nickel causes:
A. Ca lung
B. Ca nasopharynx
C. Ca ethmoid sinus
D. Ca larynx

65. Which muscle is most commonly involved in thyrotoxicosis:
A. Inferior rectus
B. Inferior oblique
C. Superior rectus
D. Superior oblique

66. Asthma mediator is a form of—
A. PGA_2
B. Prostacyclin
C. Leukotriene
D. Thromboxanes

67. Respiratory alkalosis occurs in:
A. Diabetic ketoacidosis
B. Pyloric stenosis
C. Primary aldosteronism
D. Excessive ventilation

68. Most common cause of hypercalcemic crisis is:
A. Parathyroid adenoma
B. CA Breast
C. Parathyroid hyperplasia
D. Pagets disease

69. A common cause of Cushing's syndrome is:
A. Pituitary adenoma
B. Ectopic ACTH productivity by CA
C. Adrenal Koch's
D. None of the above

70. The normal adult CSF pressure is:
A. 1-2 mm Hg
B. 6-12 mm Hg
C. 15-30 mm Hg
D. 735 mm Hg

71. Respiratory acidosis is characterized by:
A. ↓ plasma HCO3 and ↓ pCO_2
B. ↑pCO_2 and ↓ pH
C. ↓ pH and ↓ PCO_2
D. ↑pCO_2 and ↑ pH

72. Least common site for infective endocarditis:
A. ASD
B. VSD
C. Aortic Stenosis
D. Mitral stenosis

73. Autoimmune hemolytic anemia is most common in which type of Leukemia:

A. AML
B. CLL
C. Multiple myeloma
D. Sickle cell anemia

74. Perioral rash, gonadal atrophy, pigmentation in skin creases and neuritis are seen in deficiency of:

A. Zn
B. Mg
C. Selenium
D. Cobalt

75. Motor neuron disease is:

A. Involvement of anterior and lateral columns of spinal cord
B. Sensory involvement
C. Intellectual impairment
D. Ocular motility impaired

76. Commonest complication of mumps is:

A. Meningoencephalitis
B. Orchitis
C. Nerve deafness
D. Polyarthritis

77. Pulsus bisferiens is best felt in:

A. Carotid
B. Femoral
C. Radial
D. Brachial

78. Immediate treatment of peripheral circulatory failure in dengue shock syndrome is:

A. I/V high dose of dexamethasone
B. I/V crystalloid infusion
C. I/V dextrose saline
D. Dopamine + dobutamine

79. Least common site for vegetation is:

A. MS
B. AS
C. MR
D. ASD

80. Arterial blood gas analysis in carbon monoxide poisoning is:

A. PO_2 normal, O_2 saturation less
B. PO_2 less , O_2 saturation normal
C. PO_2, , O_2 saturation both decreased
D. PO_2, O_2 saturation both normal

81. Commonest chromosomal syndrome is:

A. Trisomy 13
B. Trisomy 17
C. Trisomy 21
D. Fragile x syndrome

82. What is the major change in blood vessels in hypertension:

A. Hyaline arteriosclerosis
B. Atherosclerosis
C. Multiple small aneurysms
D. Fibrinoid necrosis

83. Embolism of posterior cerebral artery leads to memory impairment because of damage to:

A. Hippocampal gyrus
B. Angular gyrus
C. Premarginal area
D. Superior temporal gyrus

84. Auto immune destruction of platelets seen in:

A. Rheumatoid arthritis
B. SLE
C. Reiter's disease
D. Polyarteritis nodosa

85. Bronchiectasis is commonest in:

A. Right middle lobe
B. Right upper lobe

C. Left lower lobe
D. Left upper lobe

86. Antihypertensive agent of choice in diabetic patient with proteinuria;
A. Enalapril
B. Clonidine
C. Alpha methyldopa
D. Propranolol

87. Endocarditis is commonest in:
A. MR
B. AS
C. Venous bypass graft
D. PDA

88. Diagnostic of RHD is:
A. Aschoff's nodule
B. MacCallum patch
C. Bread butter pericarditis
D. Shaggy vegetations

89. Tertiary parathyroidism is due to:
A. Autonomy in functioning
B. CRF
C. Adenoma
D. Malabsorption syndrome

90. Vitamin B_{12} deficiency causes:
A. Haemorrhage
B. CNS affected
C. Fits
D. Depression

91. In zinc deficiency, which of the following is not seen:
A. Acrodermatitis
B. Hypogonadism
C. Decreased wound healing
D. Goitre

92. Least common site for vegetation is:
A. MS
B. AS
C. MR
D. ASD

93. Endocarditis is commonest in:
A. MR
B. LDH
C. Venous bypass graft
D. PDA

94. Characteristic of Rheumatic / Infective endocarditis vegetations do not include:
A. Friable large vegetations on valve leaflets
B. Valve perforation
C. Myocardial absorption
D. LA thrombus

95. Region of spine most commonly affected in rheumatoid arthritis:
A. Cervical
B. Thoracic
C. Lumbar
D. Sacral

96. Which is not seen in myasthenia gravis:
A. Proximal involvement
B. ↑ In symptoms on exertion
C. Remissions occur
D. Absent DTR

97. Earliest sensation lost in diabetic neuropathy:
A. Pain
B. Temperature
C. Vibration
D. Weakness of small muscles of hand

98. Following are associated with malignancy except:
A. Down syndrome
B. Fragile X-syndrome

C. Bloom syndrome
D. Fanconi anemia

99. Acute attack of migraine is best abolished by:
A. Ergotamine
B. Sumitriptan
C. Propranolol
D. Amitriptyline

100. Alcohol damage is detected by:
A. GGT
B. SGOT
C. SGPT
D. Alk. Phosphatase

101. Weight gain is seen in following except:
A. Pheochromocytoma
B. Cushing syndrome
C. Hypothyroidism
D. Hypersecretion of insulin

102. Least common cause of infective endocarditis:
A. ASD
B. MVP
C. PDA
D. VSD

103. PCT proximal convoluteo tubular necrosis is seen in:
A. Phenol poisoning
B. Arsenic poisoning
C. Aconite poisoning
D. Lead poisoning

104. Most common presentation of primary Hyperparathyroidism is:
A. Gall stones
B. Subtle neurological and Psychiatric symptoms
C. Abdominal pain
D. Recurrent abortion

105. Most characteristic CNS lesion of HIV is:
A. Perivascular Giant cells

B. Vasculitis
C. Spongiform degeneration
D. Microglial nodules

106. Hypokalemia occurs in:
A. Meningitis
B. Hepatitis
C. Osteomyelitis
D. Bronchiolitis

107. Side effect of Zidovudine in AIDS patients is:
A. Megaloblastic anemia
B. Hyperuricemia
C. Nephrocalcinosis
D. Pancreatitis

108. Type I (IDDM) DM patient (42 years male) presenting with unilateral offensive discharge per nose. O / E, black mass is seen; the diagnosis is:
A. Inferior Turbinate atrophy
B. Mucormycosis
C. Midline lethal granuloma
D. Angiofibroma

109. To differentiate, proximal from distal renal tubular acidosis, what is used:
A. Urine pH
B. Urine aminoacids
C. Urine glucose
D. HCO_3 - levels

110. Interferon is not used in?
A. CML
B. Polymyositis
C. Hairy cell leukaemia
D. Chronic Hepatitis C infection

111. Hodgkin's lymphoma with best prognosis is:
A. Nodular sclerosing
B. Lymphocyte predominant
C. Lymphocyte depleted
D. Mixed cellularity

112. In nephritic syndrome, levels of following serum proteins decrease except:

A. Albumin
B. Fibrinogen
C. Transferrin
D. Ceruloplasmin

Answer Key to MCQs in General Medicine Part I

1	C	2	D	3	A	4	B
5	A	6	C	7	C	8	B
9	C	10	D	11	A	12	C
13	C	14	A	15	B	16	C
17	E	18	C	19	A	20	B
21	B	22	D	23	C	24	C
25	D	26	A	27	C	28	A
29	C	30	B	31	A	32	A
33	B	34	B	35	A	36	C
37	C	38	D	39	C	40	D
41	B	42	B	43	B	44	B
45	A	46	C	47	B	48	B
49	A	50	D	51	B	52	A
53	D	54	D	55	B	56	B
57	A	58	B	59	C	60	C
61	A	62	D	63	C	64	B
65	B	66	C	67	D	68	C
69	A	70	B	71	B	72	A
73	B	74	A	75	A	76	B
77	A	78	C	79	D	80	A
81	C	82	A	83	A	84	B
85	C	86	A	87	A	88	A
89	A	90	B	91	D	92	D
93	A	94	C	95	A	96	D
97	C	98	B	99	B	100	A
101	A	102	A	103	A	104	B
105	D	106	A	107	A	108	B
109	A	110	B	111	B	112	B

Part II

1. **BCG vaccine should be used within how much time after preparation:**
   A. 1 day
   B. 2 days
   C. 3 days
   D. 4 days
2. **Drug resistance is produced most commonly by which of the following antituberculous drug ?**
   A. INH
   B. Rifampicin
   C. Ethionamide
   D. Streptomycin
3. **The metabolite which accumulates in blood, in epidemic dropsy, is :**
   A. Acetic acid
   B. Pyruvic acid
   C. Acetaldehyde
   D. Formaldehyde
4. **Hepatitis virus A can be killed by:**
   A. Ultraviolet light
   B. Formalin 1 : 4000
   C. Boiling at 1000° C for 5 minutes
   D. Chlorination at 2 ppm
5. **Which of the following statement is not true about sabin vaccine**
   A. 3 doses given
   B. Given by intramuscular route
   C. Given at monthly interval
   D. Contain 3 viral strains
6. **All of the following is/are true about measles vaccine except:**
   A. Not given if history of allergy to egg
   B. Live attenuated vaccine

C. Given within one hour of reconstitution
D. Stored at 2°–10° C in a refrigerator

7. Most common method of detecting malnutrition by a health guide is:
A. Height
B. Weight
C. Mid-arm circumference
D. Skin fold thickness

8. Cereals lack which of the following amino acid:
A. Methionine
B. Lysine
C. Leucine
D. Phenylalanine

9. The protein content of cow's milk is
A. 1.2 gm%
B. 2.4 gm%
C. 3.5 gm%
D. 4.2 gm%

10. Vitamin A prophylaxis to be given 6 monthly is :
A. 6 μg
B. 66 μg
C. 6 mg
D. 66 mg

11. Which of the following is a dependent variable:
A. Cause
B. Effect
C. Association
D. Relative proportion

12. Disinfectants kill which of the following:
A. Microorganism
B. Pathogenic microorganism
C. Nonpathogenic microorganism
D. Viruses and fungi

13. Most common cause of neonatal deaths in India is :
A. Prematurity

B. Congenital malformation
C. Metabolic disease
D. Malnutrition

14. Incidence can be defined as :
A. Number of cases exiting at a given moment
B. Number of cases existing in a given population over a given period
C. Number new cases occurring during a specified period in a given population
D. Number of old cases present doing a specified period in a given population.

15. The community development programme is meant:
A. To bring about a Social and Economic change in village life through the effort of villagers themselves
B. To arrange welfare programme for women and children
C. To improve the agriculture product through better manure and seeds
D. To plan development programmers in about 100 villages with a population of about six to eight thousand.

16. The best method of health instruction is :
A. Providing reading assignment
B. Giving lectures
C. Setting example
D. Organizing film shows

17. The best teaching opportunity for a health worker in the community is while.
A. Giving health talk at home
B. Demonstrating to a group of mothers
C. Examining mother and children
D. Completing the records

18. Breast feeding is best for the baby:
A. But has no effect on the mother
B. But is likely to affect the mother's appearances adversely
C. But may cause Breast cancer in the mother
D. And is also good for the mother

19. Kwashiorkor is characterized by all of the following except
A. Apathy
B. Liver changes
C. Decreased body weight
D. Flag sign

20. Quarantine is the:
A. Minimum incubation period
B. Maximum incubation period
C. Period of infectivity
D. Serial interval

21. Cholera vaccine gives protection for:
A. 1-3 months
B. 3-6 months
C. 6-12 months
D. 12-18 months

22. Incubation period of mumps is:
A. 7 days
B. 7-14 days
C. 14-21 days
D. 21-30 days

23. Which of the following is a milk born disease:
A. Q-fever
B. Leptospirosis
C. Brucellosis
D. All of the above

24. Prevalence is calculated in a population by :
A. Finding the susceptible
B. Follow up
C. Studying cohorts
D. Studying the records

25. Correct nutritional status is best assessed by which of the following:
A. Weight for age
B. Height for age

C. Weight for height
D. Anthropometrics

26. Vi antigen of Salmonella is found to know the :
A. Carrier stage
B. Diseased stage
C. Infectivity
D. Immunity

27. For investigating an epidemic, all of the following are done except:
A. Confirmation of epidemic
B. Isolation of cases
C. Studying cofactors
D. Verification of case

28. What is the Role of Glucose in anti-diarrhoeal solution it:
A. Change taste
B. Increases absorption of sodium
C. Increases absorption of amino acids
D. Rapidly controls diarrhea by absorption of water

29. In a patient with burns more than 40%, average energy requirement in calories is:
A. 4000
B. 4500
C. 6000
D. 7000

30. Commonest cancer in males in India is of:
A. Bronchus
B. Stomach
C. Head and neck area
D. Urinary bladder

31. Appropriate fluoride levels in water in India is suggested to be:
A. 0.4 meq/L
B. 0.8 meq/L
C. 1.0 meq/L
D. 1.6 meq/L

32. Pellagra because of Jowar occurs due to:
A. High level of leucine
B. Low level of tryptophan
C. Increase in level of tryptophan
D. Low level of leonine

33. Chlorine available in fresh bleaching power is :
A. 20 %
B. 25 %
C. 33 %
D. 40 %

34. Man is intermediate host for:
A. Enterobiasis
B. Schistosomiasis haematobium
C. Taenia saginata
D. Echinococcus

35. Which of the following is a live vaccine
A. TAB
B. BCG
C. Diphtheria
D. DPT
E. Meningococcal

36. Newborn baby of a mother who had measles, is immune to this disease for
A. 4 to 6 months
B. 6 to 12 months
C. 1 to 3 years
D. 3 to 6 years
E. Life

37. Breast feeding is contraindicated if mother is receiving which of the following drugs?
A. Anti thyroid drugs
B. Broad spectrum antibiotics
C. Insulin
D. Saline
E. Streptomycin

38. Lepromin test is done to find out:
A. Indicative of delayed hypersensitivity
B. Indicative of infection
C. Negative in tubercular type
D. Positive in lepromatous type

39. The best method for sterilization of disposable items is:
A. Boiling heat
B. Dry heat
C. Gamma radiation
D. Incineration

40. Highest percentage of iron is present in which of the following:
A. Egg
B. Mutton .
C. Soybean
D. Spinach

41. In a standard normal curve, mean ± 2 standard deviation covers:
A. 60 %
B. 65 %
C. 95 %
D. 99 %

42. Ringer lactate solution contains which of the following electrolytes:
A. Na^+ and Cl^-
B. Na^+; K^+ and Cl^-
C. Na^+; K^+, Cl^- and Ca_2^+
D. Na^+; K^+ and HCO_3

43. Thiamine deficiency is best diagnosed by:
A. Erythrocyte transketolase assay
B. Blood free pyruvate levels
C. Acetyl –COA levels
D. Clinical severity of disease

44. Break point chlorination means:
A. Appearance of free chlorine in water
B. Appearance of residual chlorine in water

C. Point at which organic products are not oxidized
D. Twice the requisite amount of chlorine

45. Fiber optic instruments like endoscopes should be sterilized by:
A. Formaldehyde
B. Glutaraldehyde
C. Gamma radiation
D. Cetrimide

46. Vitamin A toxicity is manifested due to:
A. Mitochondrial damage
B. Glutaraldehyde
C. Microtubular damage
D. Endoplasmic reticulum damage

47. Ear-drum may rupture above which noise level:
A. 120 db
B. 160 db
C. 80 db
D. 90 db

48. MTP act permits termination of pregnancy up to which weeks of gestation:
A. 10
B. 12
C. 20
D. 28

49. Schick test is done to indicate:
A. Immunity to tetanus
B. Susceptibility to diphtheria
C. Immunity to diphtheria
D. Sensitivity of treatment

50. The freshly prepared ORS (Oral Rehydration Solution) should not be used for;
A. 2 hours
B. 8 hours
C. 12 hours
D. 24 hours

51. The daily extra calorie requirement in first trimester of pregnancy is:
A. 50
B. 150
C. 350
D. 450

52. Richest source of niacin is:
A. Egg
B. Meat
C. Liver
D. Milk

53. Screening of disease is what type of prevention:
A. Primary
B. Secondary
C. Tertiary
D. All of the above

54. Toxoid is prepared from:
A. Exotoxin
B. Endotoxin
C. Both
D. None of the above

55. Carcinoma more prevalent in persons working in dye industry of:
A. Bones
B. Skin
C. Lungs
D. Bladder

56. Dengue spreads by:
A. Anopheles
B. Culex
C. Aedes
D. Mansoides

57. Excessive crying is seen after vaccination of:
A. BCG
B. Polio

C. DPT
D. Measles

58. Strict vegetarians are deficient in:
A. B_1
B. Biotin
C. B_{12} / cyanocobalamine
D. Vitamin D

59. Most immediate treatment of night blindness is:
A. Topical Vitamin A
B. Vitamin A orally
C. Vitamin A parenterally
D. Any of the above

60. Treatment of choice for diphtheria carrier is:
A. Erythromycin
B. Tetracycline
C. Penicillin
D. DPT

61. Spread of dispersion means:
A. Mean
B. Mode
C. Median
D. Standard deviation

62. Constituents of 'Savlon' are:
A. Cetrimide +Chlorhexidine
B. Cetrimide + quarternary ammonium compound
C. Buffered glutaraldehyde
D. Certrimide only

63. Γ- globulins do not interact with immunity of:
A. Mumps
B. Measles
C. Rubella
D. Oral polio

64. Control of reservoir for presentation of disease is done with:
A. Tetanus
B. Rabies

C. Influenza
D. Diphtheria

65. Normal distribution of a curve depends upon:
A. Mean
B. Standard deviation
C. A + B
D. Mean + Range

66. 'Confidence + Limits' are:
A. Mean +Standard error
B. Median + Standard error
C. Mean + Range
D. Mean + Standard deviations

67. Which of the following immunoglobulins is found in saliva?
A. Ig M
B. Ig A
C. Ig E
D. Ig D
E. Ig G

68. Transplacental immunity is seen in all except:
A. Diphtheria
B. Pertusis
C. Polio
D. Measles

69. Primary prevention of diabetes mellitus includes all except:
A. Reduction of weight
B. Prevent hypertension
C. Exercise
D. Avoid-excessive sweets

70. Food poisoning is caused by all except:
A. Cl. septicum
B. Cl. welchii
C. Cl. Oedematicus
D. S. typhimururium

71. The fluid requirements per kilogram of body weight are highest:

A. In the first week of the life
B. Between ages of 1 to 6 months
C. Between ages up to 24 months
D. Above the age of 24 months.

72. Measles vaccine is not given below the age of:

A. 9 months
B. 12 months
C. 15 months
D. 18 months

73. Primary chemoprophylaxis belongs to which level of prevention:

A. Ist
B. 2nd
C. 3rd
D. 4th

74. All of the following are true vaccines except:

A. Cholera
B. BCG
C. Typhoid
D. DPT

75. Which of the following cereals is richest in calcium:

A. Wheat
B. Gram
C. Rice
D. Bajra

76. Hepatitis A virus is destroyed by all except:

A. Chlorine 1 ppm
B. Boiling at 100° C for 6 min
C. UV rays
D. Formalin 1:4000

77. Terms mild, moderate and severe are which type of variable:

A. Interval
B. Nominal.

C. Ordinate
D. Ratio

78. Man is an intermediate host for:
A. P.vivax
B. Strongyloides stercorales
C. Enterobius
D. Trichiuris trichura

79. Dally requirement of calcium in pregnancy is:
A. 50 mg
B. 100 mg
C. 500 mg
D. 1000 mg

80. Herd immunity is not useful in protection against:
A. Polio
B. Diphtheria
C. Measles
D. Tetanus

81. In a patient with AIDS, can not be given all of the following vaccines except:
A. BCG
B. DPT
C. OPV
D. Measles

82. The Best Epidemoilogical marker for the HBV:
A. HBc Ag
B. HBs Ag
C. Anti HBs Ag antibody
D. HBe Ag

83. Best indicator for Hepatitis – B infection of community:
A. Hepatitis B antigen
B. Core Antigen
C. Core Antibody
D. Hepatitis B Antibody

84. Best source of vitamin B_{12} is:
A. Milk

B. Liver
C. Soyabean
D. Leafy vegetables

85. Mosquito acts as intermediate vector in:
A. Filaria
B. Cholera
C. Typhoid
D. Malaria

86. Carcinoma least amenable to screening is of:
A. Lung
B. Breast
C. Cervix
D. Oral cavity

87. Variables are arranged in ascending or descending order to find:
A. Mean
B. Median
C. Mode
D. Standard deviation

88. Which of the following is an absolute contraindication for combined oral pills:
A. Diabetes mellitus
B. Hypertension
C. Previous history of thromboembolism
D. Heart disease

89. Incidence is calculated by:
A. Prospective study
B. Retrospective study
C. Cross-sectional study
D. Random study

90. Epidemiologic study of Hepatitis B:
A. HbsAg is used
B. IgG anti HBC
C. Hb C Ag
D. HBeAg

91. Student's t - test:

A. Is used to calculate attributable risk
B. Is used to calculate relative risk
C. To find out degree of significance
D. To calculate generation time of a disease

92. Vaccine not given to immuno-competent siblings of immuno deficient children:

A. Oral polio
B. MMR
C. Measles
D. DPT

93. Additional protein requirement per day during lactation is:

A. 14 g
B. 25 g
C. 35 g
D. 45 g

94. Benzathine penicillin given in RHD is which type of prevention:

A. Primordial
B. Primary
C. Secondary
D. Tertiary

95. Which of the following is a subcutaneous vaccine:

A. Measles
B. BCG
C. DPT
D. Polio

96. Quarantine is defined as:

A. Diseased individual isolated till symptoms subside
B. Healthy individual isolated after exposure to disease
C. Healthy individual isolated before exposure to disease
D. Diseased individual isolated till no secondary case occurs

97. Vaccine contraindicated in pregnancy is:

A. Tuberculin
B. Polio

C. Hepatitis B
D. Typhoid

98. In a patient with AIDS, you do not give which vaccine:
A. BCG
B. DPT
C. OPV
D. Measles

99. Most common cancer reported in India is:
A. Ca cervix
B. Ca lung
C. Ca breast
D. Ca oral cavity

100. 'DOTS' is:
A. Short term chemotherapy under direct observation
B. Long term chemotherapy under observation
C. Long term chemotherapy without supervision
D. Free drug distribution to patients

101. Quarantine is:
A. To keep the patient for longest incubation period
B. To keep the patient for shortest incubation period
C. To isolate for lag period
D. To isolate for generation time

102. Additional calories required during Lactation is:
A. 450
B. 550
C. 650
D. 750

103. Normal iron requirement during pregnancy is:
A. 2 mg
B. 40 mg
C. 80 mg
D. 100 mg

104. Active & Passive immunity is given simultaneously for the following except:
A. Hepatitis B

B. Tetanus
C. Measles
D. Rabies

105. Vitamin D is not present in:
A. Milk
B. Fish fat
C. Cod liver oil
D. Egg

106. Amount of weight gain per unit quantity protein is:
A. Protein efficiency ratio
B. Net protein utilization
C. Biological value
D. Digestibility coefficient

Answer Key to MCQs in General Medicine Part II

1	A	2	A	3	B	4	C
5	C	6	D	7	C	8	B
9	C	10	D	11	B	12	B
13	A	14	C	15	A	16	C
17	C	18	D	19	C	20	B
21	B	22	C	23	D	24	B
25	C	26	A	27	B	28	B
29	C	30	C	31	C	32	A
33	C	34	D	35	B	36	B
37	A	38	A	39	C	40	B
41	C	42	C	43	B	44	A
45	B	46	A	47	A	48	C
49	B	50	D	51	B	52	B
53	B	54	A	55	D	56	C
57	C	58	C	59	B	60	A
61	D	62	A	63	D	64	B
65	C	66	A	67	B	68	B
69	A	70	C	71	B	72	A
73	A	74	D	75	D	76	A
77	A	78	A	79	D	80	D
81	B	82	A	83	B	84	B
85	A	86	A	87	B	88	C
89	A	90	B	91	C	92	A
93	B	94	C	95	A	96	B
97	A	98	D	99	D	100	A
101	A	102	B	103	B	104	C
105	A	106	A				

20

Fluorides and Community Dentistry

- Primary prevention = i.e. the steps taken to ensure disease does not occur.
- Secondary prevention = promoting early intervention in those already affected to halt progression at incipient stage of the disease.
- Tertiary prevention = Rx of well established disease to restore function and avoid further episodes.
- **Cross sectional** study = samples are different individuals at the same age intervals.
- **Experimental** study = in it, the investigator can manipulate the independent variables.
- **Double – blind** study = i.e. neither the persons collecting the data nor the people participating as subjects will not know all the details of the study.
- **Longitudinal** study = serial studies of same individual over a period of time.
- **Single blind** study = only the investigator, but not the subjects, know which is the drug under study.
- Measures of **central tendency** = mean; median; mode.
- Measures of **dispersion** = range; mean deviation; standard deviation; variance; probability.
- When disease spreads from man to animals is ka = zoo anthroposes.

- TRIPLE BLIND STUDY—ie data collection, subjects and analyses will not known anything about the study.
- When disease spreads from animal to man is ka = **anthropozoonoses**.
- When disease spreads either way is ka = **amphixenosis**
- **Exotic** refers the disease imported into the country.
- **Epizootic** refers to epidemic disease occurring in animals.
- **Public health** is defined as art and science of preventing disease, prolonging life, and promoting physical and mental efficiency through organized community efforts.

Normal distribution curve = it can be expressed as below in terms of mean and SD which in turn will depend upon number and nature of observations.

- It is a smooth bell shaped curve.
- It is symmetrical and has height frequency in middle;
- The frequency goes on decreasing on either side.

STANDARD NORMAL CURVE

- Total area of curve = 1
- Standard deviation = 1
- Mean = 0
- Mean = median = mode
- The distance of a value (X) from the mean of curvature in units of SD is ka relative deviate standard normal variate.
- There are no boundaries in either direction, for the curve never touches the base line, no matter how far it extends.
- Curve is the curve of probability, not the certainty.
- The area b/w one SD on either side of the mean = 68.3% (± 1 S.D)
- The area b/w 2 SD on either side of the mean = 95.4% (± 2 S.D)
- The area b/w 3 SD on either side of the mean = 99.7% (± 3 S.D)
- It is artifically designed by the statistician for the sample to be covered in the total area.

Chi – square test

- Statistical measure used in context of sampling analysis for comparing variance to a theoretical variance.

- Method of comparing experimentally obtained results with those to be expected theoretically on some hypothesis.
- It is used to found significance of 2 or more than 2 proportions.
- It is used as a test of association b/w 2 events in binomial or multinomial samples.

T – test

- It is an appropriate test for judging the significance **of a sample mean.**
- For judging the significance of **difference between the means** of 2 samples.
- It can also be used for judging the significance of coefficients of simple and partial correlations.

Correlation

- To find out whether there **is association between 2 variables**, we calculate coeff of correlation (*r*).
- It tends to be b/w –1.0 to + 1.0
- If it is near to + 1 == it shows strong +ve correlation b/w 2 variables, i.e. if one increases, the other will also increase.
- If it is near – 1 == it shows strong – ve correlation, i.e. if one increases, the other decreases.
- If r = 0, there is no correlation.

Regression

Change in measurements of a variable character on the positive or negative test.

- Children dental health week = first week in February
- Bar diagram = used only one variable; **qualitative** data;

OHI index (OHI-S) = measures the oral hygiene; teeth selected are = 6, 1 / 6 in upper arch; and 6 /1, 6 in lower arch, i.e. max first molars and right CI; and mand first molars and left CI.

- Labial surface of upper and lower CI; and Buccal surface of upper molars, i.e. of 11, 16, 26, 31 teeth
- Lingual surface of lower molars, i.e. 36, 46 teeth.

- **Tip** thickness of **Moller's index** is 18 microns.
- **Ramfjord's index**, the teeth examined are = 6/1, 4 in upper arch; 4, 1/6 in lower arch.
- The modified **navy plaque index** divided each tooth surface into 9 areas of the 6 index teeth used by Ramfjord.
- Disclosing agent in modified **Quigley Hein plaque index** is basic fuschin.
- Most commonly used disclosing agent is = **erythrosin.**

FLUORIDES

1. FLUOROSIS / MOTTLING = aka **Colorado stains**; found by McKay 1901
2. Shoe – leather survey = by T H Dean in 1933 – 34
3. Dean and his coworkers 1920 – 1936 found that water with 1 ppm F had a maximum cariostatic effect.
4. Tea leaves contain 98 ppm F.
5. 1 ppm = 1 gm / 1000 litres = 1 mg / litre
6. First artificial water fluoridation = in Grands Rapids in 1945. Grand Rapids was the subject; muskegon was the control.
7. F – plasma levels = 19 – 38 ng / ml
8. F water levels according to **atmospheric temperature** should be –
   a. in hot = 0.7 ppm
   b. moderate = 1.0 ppm
   c. cold = 1.2 ppm
9. 0.7 - 1.2 ppm level is caries preventive; is the range.
10. F is mainly excreted by KIDNEYS.
11. Locally applied F is more effective than systemic F.
12. F forms **fluorhydroxyapatite crystals** and make enamel resistant to acids.
13. 32 ppm F is required in plaque to decrease acid production.
14. FLUORIDIZATION = it is the process of topical application of F to the teeth, as given by **Bibby in 1941.**

15. KNUTSON'S TECHNIQUE = topical application of 2 % NaF for 4 min every week for 4 weeks; done 4 times / year at 3, 7, 10, and 13 years of age (i.e. a total of 64 visits).
16. F is absorbed by PASSIVE DIFFUSION in GIT.
17. Oral lethal dose of F = 2 – 3 gm. 5 mg/kg body wt. is the potentially ORAL LETHAL DOSE.
18. Largest amount of NaF tab prescribed at any time according to ADA specification = 120 tabs of 2.2 mg each = 264 mg.
19. I tab NaF of 2.2 mg = 1.0 mg F
20. F concentration in blood, saliva and soft tissues = 0.1 ppm
21. % age of F in tooth paste = 1000 ppm
22. 95 % of total body F is in hard tissues.
23. Highest calcified tissue conc of F is in = cementum.
24. Enamel formed under 1 ppm F level of water has about = 1000 – 2000 ppm F in its outermost layers, i.e. 1 – 2 microns thickness.
25. 8% SnF_2 is used for topical application for 4 min, once a year.
26. SnF_2 is 3 times more effective than NaF.
27. 1.23% APF is 1.5 × more effective than NaF.
28. BRUDEVOLD'S SOLUTION = is 1.23% APF.
29. Organic F, e.g. amine fluorides are better than inorganic F.
30. F mouth rinses should be started after = 6 yrs age.
31. Best effect is achieved when F is ingested systemically during MINERALISATION of surface of crown.
32. F inhibits enz ENOLASE of glycolysis and so prevents acid formation.
33. F doses

Age yrs	**Dose, mg / day**
0 – 2	0.25 / upto 0.5 mg
2 – 3	0.5 / upto 0.5 – 0.7 mg
3 – 12	1.0 / 1.0 – 1.5 mg

RECOMMENDED USE of F toothpaste

34. **Use** of F pastes

Age yrs	**Summary**	**Advise**
0 – 4	No F	Brushing twice a day without paste
4 – 6	1 F + 2 non-F	Brushing once daily with F paste and 2 times without paste
6 – 8	2 F + 1 non-F	Twice daily with F paste and once without any paste
> 8	3 F	Brush thrice daily with F paste

35. F supplementations

F water levels → Age of the child ↓	0 – 0.3 ppm	0.3 – 0.7 ppm	> 0.7 ppm	Summary
0 – 2 yrs	0.25 mg	0 mg	0 mg	¼ mg
2 – 3 yrs	0.5 mg	0.25 mg	0 mg	½ mg
> 3 yrs	1.0 mg	0.5 mg	0 mg	1 mg

36. Why deciduous teeth do not show mottling ? = because primary teeth have a short pre-eruptive maturation period.
37. 2.2 mg tab of NaF gives 1 mg of F; similarly 1.1 mg tab of NaF gives 0.50 mg of F; and 0.5 mg tab gives 0.25 mg of F.
38. F is stored in plaque and on enamel surface as CaF_2 – like precipitate.
39. F helps remineralisation of <u>white spot lesions</u> only if surface of enamel is intact.
40. For F mouth-rinses
    - use 0.05 % NaF daily
    - or 0.2 % NaF fortnightly
    - or 0.02 % APF daily
    - or 0.2 % APF fortnightly
    - or 0.025 % NaF daily, in the fluoridated areas.

41. F dentifrices = NaMFP is better than NaF, SnF_2.
42. For children less than 4 years age = F paste is not recommended.
43. DEAN'S INDEX for Fluorosis –

Normal	0	Enamel translucent; surface smooth, glossy
Questionable	0.5	– Slight aberrations from normal – few white flecks to occasional white spots
Very mild	1	– small, opaque, paper white areas not involving > 25% of tooth surface
Mild	2	– White opaque areas on enamel not involving > 50% surface
Moderate	3	– All enamel surfaces affected – Increased wear – Brown stains
Severe	4	– Enamel hypoplasia – Discrete or confluent pitting – Widely spread brown stains – Teeth representing CORRODED-APPEARANCE

IMPORTANT POINTS

- F is among 14 trace elements which are physiologically essential for normal growth and development.
- F is not found in free elemental form in nature and appears rather as compound F because of its **most electronegative nature**.
- It is the 13th most common element in earth crust.
- F is readily absorbed from stomach and also from skin and lungs.
- Maximum plasma conc., i.e. 0.15 – 0.25 ppm is reached within 60 min.

- At 1 ppm = there is **60 % reduction in caries rate.**

  F is found in the form of
  - Fluorspar / fluorite = CaF_2
  - Fluorapatite = $Ca_3\ (PO_4)_2.\ F_2$
  - Cryolite = $Na_3\ AlF_6$.
- In INDIA, on an average, by age of 15 yrs, the DMFT is 3.
- According to WHO, the DMFT of 2 by 15 yrs should cause the alarm.
- In India, the dentist – population ratio = 1 : 80,000
- In USA, ideal ratio should be = 1 : 2,000.

  In India, the population lives in
  - Endemic area = 5 %
  - Optimal F area = 3 %
  - Fluoride deficient area = 85 – 90 %
- In 1901, Dr. Fredick Mckay of Colorade / USA found many of his patients had permanent stains on teeth = ka COLORADO STAINS, McKay called it the **mottled enamel.**
- **Denti di chiaic** = Dr. JM Eager, reported ugly brown stains on the teeth of residents of Naples.
- Epidemiologic studies have shown that fluoridation of water supply not only reduces the occurrence of caries but also affects a significant reduction of incidence of periodontal disease.
- **Reverse swallowing habits** are extremely difficult to correct and involve a combination of muscle exercise and appliances as well as psychological counselling.
- Fluoride taken systemically is **excreted in urine** and deposited in fingernails and toenails. It is also deposited in teeth and bone. Almost, 20–30% is excreted in urine within 3 – 4 hrs.
- **Fluoride content** of = cementum > bone > dentin > enamel (CBDE); In calculus, mineral is equivalent to the dentin.
- Maximum F is found in = cementum
- Lethal dose of F = 32 – 64 mg / kg wt
- Safe toxic dose of F = $1/4^{th}$ of LD, i.e. 8 – 16 mg / kg wt
- 1 mg of F = 2.2 mg of NaF ; 1 drop = 0.1 ppm

- **Most effective method** of preventing the dental decay in population is = systemic fluorides.
- F is mainly removed by the body in URINE.
- F is absorbed from stomach; lungs and rarely from skin.

  F content in
  - Fish = dried mackerel = 84.9 ppm
  - In dried salmon = 19.3 ppm
  - In tea leaves = 97.0 ppm
  - In potato = 6.4 ppm

- **Metallic taste** after application of **stannous fluoride** is due to the formation of tin hydroxyphosphate.
- The amount of F^- present in the **outermost surface of enamel** under the influence of 1 ppm in drinking water is = 1000 – 2000 ppm.

- Amount of water consumption increases during the warmer climate. So F-should be less in water.
- In cold climate, the recommended F level may be as high as 1.2 ppm, because less water is consumed in cold weathers.
- Extremely hot climates, a level of about 0.7 ppm is OK, because more water is consumed.
- Moderately warm climate = 1 ppm.

- Ppm F = 0.34 / E where E = - 0.038 + 0.0062 x T (in F).
- McKay showed that there is **inverse relation** b/w incidence of very mild mottling and dental caries.
- NaF mouth rinse allowed in fluoridated area = 0.025 % NaF solution weekly/fortnightly.
- NaF mouth rinse allowed in non - fluoridated area = 0.05 % NaF solution daily.
- **Disclosing agent** in modified Quigley Hein plaque index = **basic fuschin.**
- **Xylitol** can be used as a **sugar substitute** in processed food.
- F levels per gram dry wt of plaque are = 13 – 55 microgram.
- In comparison to normal enamel, the **carious enamel will take up fluoride faster**.

- Probing pressure in CPITN is = 20 gms
- A therapeutic vitamin would have dosage of nutrients greater than recommended dietary allowance by = 5 – 10 times.
- After tooth cleaning, the new plaque growth originates from the gingival sulcus.
- According to the Stephen curve, the **raw starch is least cariogenic**.
- In plaque = IgG and IgA are found.
- **Engerix – B** against hepatitis B virus is an example of active immunity and **recombinant DNA vaccine.**
- In Breast milk, F will be 6 – 12 micro gm /ml.
- Upon acid attack, F will enter the tooth in HF form.
- Primary purpose of OHI – S index is = to assess the debris and calculus; a useful tool in studying the relationship b/w periodontitis and oral cleanliness.
- OHI – S index = is **reversible index**
- Russell periodontal index = reversible as well as irreversible index.
- Hypothetical optimum dentist to population ratio is = 1 : 2000

Primary function of delta dental plans is

- To act as an advisory group to ADA.
- To act as an advisory group to practising dentist.
- To create a vehicle through which individual service plans could participate in underwriting contacts from different states.

Effect of levels of fluoride

1.	0.7 – 1.2 ppm	normal
2.	1.5 – 3.0 ppm for 5 – 10 yrs age old child	mild fluorosis/dental
3.	4.0 – 8.0 ppm for > 10 yrs	severe dental fluorosis/mild skeletal fluorosis
4.	more than 8 ppm for 5 – 10 yrs age	severe dental and skeletal fluorosis

- Systemically fluoridation or artificial fluoridation of community water reduces caries by 60 %.
- The **ameloblasts** in developing enamel show a **selective response** to the introduction of NaF and are disturbed and **become inflammed** when high levels of fluorides are ingested.
- Dry heat sterilisation is better for sharp instruments while steam sterilisation try to dull the sharp instruments.
- The most common cause of gingival enlargement is = inflammation.
- Chronic gingivitis can be seen as early as 5 yrs of age.

PITS AND FISSURE SEALANTS

- Best age for application of pit and fissure sealants is = b/w 6 – 12 yrs age; because this is age in which P and F of permanent teeth get decayed. Enamel etched by tooth conditioners but not covered by fissure sealants **will remineralise with in a week.**
- The fissure sealants will not stay on the teeth if the surfaces are shiny when sealant is applied, i.e. if the surface is not dry or if it is wet.
- Retention of fissure sealants is **greater in permanent teeth** than the primary teeth and about 50 % in primary teeth after 2 yrs age.

- CO_2 lasers are use for **fissure sealing**.
- First generation sealants = activated by UV light.
- 2nd generation sealants = chemical curing resins.
- 3rd generation sealants = activated by visible light.
- F containing sealants = give double protections.

- 90 mg F / **kg salt** initially in Switzerland reduced **20 –25 % caries** rate.
- 2.5 mg NaF in addition *to milk* reduced caries by *36.3 %.*
- For 50 % caries reduction, only **0.25 rupees/year/individual expenditure** occurs.
- Cost – benefit ratio = 1 : 160
- The fluoride and hydroxyl has primary hydration no. = 5

- And ionic radii of F = 1.29 Å; of OH^- = 1.33 Å.
- The isomorphic replacement of OH – ions by F ions brings about very slight shortening of 'a' axis of hydroxyapatite crystals from 9.42 Å to 9.37 Å. and 'o' axis remains unchanged.
- The amount of F needed to replace all the hydroxyls of HA is 2 % unit cells.
- Enamel formed under the influence of 1 ppm F in drinking water has about 1000 to 2000 ppm in outermost layer.
- The conversion of HA to fluorapatite is only = 3 – 5 %
- Small amount of F ions, 1–10 ppm will **reduce the acid production** by pure culture on saliva glucose mixture.
- Higher levels of ionic F, above the 32 ppm are required to reduce acid production by plaque.
- **0.2 % of chlorohexidine** = causes total inhibition of new plaque formation.
- Zn – citrate = 0.2 % twice a day; helps in plaque inhibition.
- Semitronic tooth brush gives = 520 strokes / second

BIBBY TECHNIQUE = of topical application of NaF is

- 0.1 % NaF solution.
- 7 min. application
- 3 times / year in 1st year = at 4 mos. Interval.
- 6 times / yr – in 2nd yr = at 2 months interval.
- 45 % decrease in caries in = 1st yr
- 33 % decrease in caries in = 2nd yr
- 36 % decrease in caries in = 3rd yr

KNUTSON'S TECHNIQUE

- 2 % NaF solution
- 20 gm / litre
- at the age of **3,7,10,13 yrs** because at these ages, the new teeth erupt.
- 4 times weekly interval
- total no. of patient's visits = 64, i.e. (One visit/wk for 4 weeks; repeated after **every 3 months interval**; at the ages specified, i.e. 3,7,10,13 yrs).

- Decrease in caries = 39.8 %.
- Disadvantage = patient must take multiple visits to dentist.
- After application, do not rinse with water for upto 30 min.
- It should not be stored in glass bottles due to formation of Si F_2.

SnF 2 = 8 % solution; there is 2 % F in it .

- PH of freshly prepared solution = 2.5
- Usually applied **once a year.**
- It should be freshly prepared.
- It reduces caries by 80 %.
- It does not etch porcelain.
- Antimicrobial and antiplaque properties.
- Can be used in adults.
- **Metallic taste** due to formation of tin-hydroxyphosphate.
- Gingival blanching.
- **Stains** the silicate and composite resins.
- Causes **artifacts on R/G**.
- Stannide capsule contains 800 mg of SnF_2.
- Enamel is least perfectly remineralised.

APF GEL / ACIDULATED phosphate flouride

- Topical F **most commonly used** in dental offices
- 1.23 % conc / 12300 ppm; aka **Brudevold's solution.**
- PH = 3.0
- Gels are **thixotropic** and flows easily into interproximal spaces.
- In gels, the gelling agent is **methyl cellulose** or hydroxy ethyl cellulose; the pH is 4 – 5.
- It is usually **applied semiannually.**
- It etches the porcelain restorations.

VARNISHES = **semiannually** application;

Main advantage of F varnish is **prolonged contact** and penetration into tooth enamel.

Duraphet is NaF varnish, 2.26 % = 22600 ppm.

Fluoro-protector is silane fluoride ; 0.7 %.

0.3 – 0.5 ml of varnish equal to 6.9 – 11.5 mg of F is required to cover full dentition.

Never isolate with cotton during application with fluorides.

Main drawback is restriction of diet.

Fluorosis normally does not occur in primary teeth but can occur at 15 ppm of water – F conc; because primary teeth are exposed to fluoride for a short interval only during calcification.

Methods of school F programme

- School water fluoridation = 4.5 ppm
- **Weekly rinse** with 0.2 % NaF
- 1 mg of F daily
- 4 minutes of daily application of gels in tray
- Topical application of F on yearly basis.
- School water fluoridation is 20 % less than the community water fluoridation.

Fluoride mouth rinses = (daily = 0.05 % NaF); (weekly/ fortnightly = 0.2 %)

- Frequent use of low conc of F for topical application is more cariostatic than less frequent use of higher conc of topical application.
- Daily rinsing of 0.05 % of NaF, i.e. 225 ppm + 0.2% weekly/ fortnightly in school in non-fluoridated areas.
- For superadded benefit, 0.025% NaF solution weekly / fortnightly.
- Mouth rinses used mainly in patients *with rampant caries.*
- In cases of Reduced salivary flow, daily use is recommended.
- In handicapped persons.

FLUORIDE TABLETS = fluoraday, tymafluor; luride tabs.

- Both systemic and topical actions.
- Tablets are chewed, swished and swallowed.

- Usually not recommended below 18 mos. of age and after 13 yrs of age.
- 1 tab of 2.2 mg of NaF produce 1 mg of active F.
- It is considered to dispense 120 mg of F / 240 mg of NaF at a time.
- Dose is dependent on age and conc. of F in water.

Other imp points

- F effects are always *additive.*
- Multiple F therapy is always beneficial.
- Mostly recommended or widely used in dentrifrices now is **sodium mono fluoro phosphate (SMFP).**
- **Nalgonda technique** uses = lime; bleaching powder; filter alum.
- F levels = 13 – 55 micro gm of dry wt of plaque.
- Newly erupted teeth has high affinity for F.
- Breast milk has = 6 – 12 micro gm of F conc.
- **Accretion** = i.e. F is buried within the mineral crystallites at time of crystal growth.
- Fluoride content in bone = is more in cancellous bone; increased with age; reaches with plateau by age 55 yrs.
- F **partially crosses the placenta in** late stages. Recent concept is that placenta is not a barrier AT ALL for the fluoride.
- Saliva has = 0.01 – 0.03 ppm
- Starch is usually not broken down in the oral cavity to become a significant source of bacterial nutrition.
- Starch is least cariogenic.
- High carbohydrate food is the most frequent cause of dental decay in primary teeth.
- When the first permanent teeth begin to erupt, the prevalence of dental decay in primary teeth is approx 80 %.
- In preschool children, about 50 % decay is there.
- **Unwaxed thin dental floss** is the most preferred floss.

- Gingivitis appears within 1 week if oral hygiene is neglected.
- Maturation of plaque is often associated with mineralization, this process normally begins at the tooth surface and **proceeds outwards**, ultimately producing dense calculus and important etiologic agent in the PDL diseases. Outermost layer of plaque is thus soft and non – mineralised, the recent layer.

Optimum temperature for culturing the most microbes causing human disease is 37° C.

Tooth brushing techniques = tooth brushing is most effective in preventing the PD diseases.

- **Bass** = a good method for cleaning of **sulcus;** stimulates the gingiva.
- **Side to side** = a method is **destructive** to both hard and soft tissues.
- **Roll stroke** = tooth brushing method **least likely to remove plaque** in gingival margin.
- A disclosing wafer is useful in evaluating efficiency of tooth brushing.
- Best **disclosing agent** is = 1 – 3 tetrazolium compound with **methylene blue**. It stains only plaque.
- First modern tooth brush was invented by chinese.
- Most effective method of tooth brushing is = 5 – in – 1 method;
- Most bristles of a battery-driven tooth brush are = **vertical direction**.

Differences b/w Snyder and LA colony count tests

Property	**Snyder test**	**LA colony count**
Incubation temp	37° C	37° C
Incubation period	72 hrs	96 hrs
Method of reading test	Colorimetric	Colony count
Culture medium	Glucose agar	Tomato agar
Method of incubation	Incubator	Incubator

ON CARIES

- Hopewood House study = in Australia; in institutionalized young children; **sucrose** was the agent used.
- Turku study by Makinen = sucrose was replaced by **xylitol** as the agent.
- **Vipeholm study** = on **mentally defective patients; sucrose** was used; it concluded that physical form of carbohydrate is much more important in cariogenicity than total amount of sugar ingested. It is the most unethical study.
- Caloric sweeteners = polyalcohol; sorbitol; xylitol.
- Low caloric sweeteners = aspartase; saccharin; cyclamate.
- Chlorhexidine = bis – guanide compound; antiseptic.
- Capacity of saliva sample to dissolve enamel is determined by = Fesdick X deewar test.
- **The use of bitewing r/g** in examinations for dental caries increases the amount of caries detected by = 20 – 50 %.
- Approx 75 % of incipient interproximal caries will be undetected in preschool children if good bite wing r/g are not used.
- **Cosmetic toothpaste** = it consists of more of abrasive agent and or either bleaching agent for whitening of tooth and to improve esthetics, e.g. shine and smile.
- Tobacco smoking through Hukka is least harmful.
- Buccal mucosa shows maximum malignancy rate.

Systemic fluorides = i.e. in blood; get deposited in developing teeth; also have topical effect through saliva.

Cariostatic mechanism of fluorides = rendering enamel more resistant to acid dissolution. F ions fill the voids of HA crystals due to missing – OH groups and add their H – bonding tendency to the forces which hold the crystals together and decreases the solubility.

F ions can fit perfectly in the center of triangular arrangement of Ca ions present **in HA structure** (Young and Iliot 1966 described triangular structure of HA).

So HA + F → FHA (Fluor-hydroxy apatite)

Amount of F needed to replace - OH of HA is **2 per unit cell.**

Enamel formed under the influence of 1 ppm of F in water has about **1000 – 2000 ppm F on its outermost surface**, i.e. the conversion of HA → FA is only 3 – 5 %.

Enamel which is mineralised under F has lower CO_3^- content and so **decreased solubility.**

F causes remineralisation of early carious lesions, if the enamel surface is continuous.

Enzymatic action = F inhibits acid production by **inhibiting enz enolase**. Bound F gets concentrated in plaque and keeps on releasing F ions.

F decreases transport or uptake of glucose or glucose analogues into the cells of oral streptococci.

F inhibits the metabolism of polysaccharides by the bacteria in plaque and by salivary bacteria and thus **inhibiting acid production,** dextrans and levans formation.

F in surface enamel **alters the surface charge / free energy** and so indirectly alters the deposition of pellicle and so plaque formation.

F alters tooth morphology, i.e. decreases the cusps height, fissure depth etc. making the tooth less caries susceptible.

WATER FLUORIDATION = done at 2 levels, i.e. community water fluoridation and school water fluoridation.

First community water fluoridation = done in **Grand Rapids** in USA.

Decrease in caries in primary teeth = 40 – 50 %

Decrease in caries in secondary teeth = 50 – 60 %

1 ppm F is the recommended level.

Optimum levels of F varies with **climate/temperature** as the average consumption of water increases in warmer time.

Ppm of F conc. = 0.34 / E; where E = - 0.038 + 0.0062 x temp in F.

Temp in °C	Recommended ppm levels
< 18.3	1.1 – 1.3 ppm
18.9 – 26.6	0.8 – 1.0
> 26.7	0.5 – 0.7

Compounds used in water fluoridation

1. Fluorspar = has CaF_2
2. NaF = is expensive
3. Silicofluorides
4. Sodium silicofluorides = **most popular;** produced from hydro flusilicic acid.
5. Hydroflusilicic acid
6. Ammonium silico fluoride

School water fluoridation = decreases DMFT by 40 – 50 %

Recommended levels should be 4.5 – 6.3 ppm in India.

More effective in permanent dentition by this age.

Salt fluoridation = 20 – 25 % caries reduction

First time done in 1955 in *Switzerland.*

Requires = 300 mg of F / kg of salt which gives 1.5 mg F from 15 mg of salt is safe;

NaF, CaF_2, KF can be added to the salts.

Milk fluoridation = given by Ziegler in 1956

36.3 % caries decreases with 2.5 mg NaF in milk.

Fluoride tablets

- These give systemic effects before mineralisation of the teeth and local effect thereafter by chewing.

Primary teeth = caries decrease is 50 – 80 % when the F administration is started before 2 yrs age and continued for 3 – 4 yrs.

Permanent teeth = 20 – 40 % reduction of caries; longest clinical trial by Aasenden and Peebler 1974.

Latest accepted dosage for F tablets by WHO / CDA etc.

	F in water supply		
Age of the child	< 0.3 mg / L	0.3 – 0.6 mg / L	> 0.6 mg / L
0 – 6 mos	—	—	—
> 6 mos – 3 yrs	0.25 mg / day	—	—
> 3 yrs – 6 yrs	0.5 mg / day	0.25	—
> 6 yrs	1.0 mg / day	0.5	0.25

Fluoride drops = for 16 – 18 weeks old infants;

10 drops = 1 mg of F

10 drops in 1 liter of water =1 ppm, i.e. 1 mg / liter

Food stuffs = fish = 0.5 mg / day (40 mg / kg in fish)

Maximum F is found in tea = 0.04 – 2.7 mg / day

Intake of ambient air with F conc. 0.16 mg / m^3 gives 3.2 mg of F/day to a person.

Most imp source is = fluoridated water.

Infants = human milk contains F = 6 – 12 mg / liter.

Fluoride toxicity

- **Certain lethal dose** = 32 – 64 mg / kg of body wt.
  ie 2.5 – 10 gm = adults
  4 – 5 gm = children
  0.25 gm = infants.
- **Safely tolerated dose** = 8 – 16 mg / kg of body wt.
- **Acute lethal dose** of F = 50 mg / kg of body wt.

- **Potentially lethal dose** = 14 – 28 mg / kg body wt.
- F + HCl in GIT = HF acid is formed which has **corrosive effect** on GIT mucosa.
- F poisoning causes = **hypocalcemia**, so Ca^{++} becomes indispensable for functional integrity of voluntary and ANS and may cause paraesthesia, paresis, tetany, convulsions etc.
- F poisoning causes = **hyperkalemia,** so ventricular arrythmias and cardiac arrest.
- F may interfere with enzymes having Mg, Mn, with glycolytic enz., cholinesterases.
- Concentrated F solutions (10 mg / ml) should not be prescribed so as to avoid mishaps.
- F mouth-rinses should not be given to kids < 6 yrs of age.
- 0.2% NaF solution wk/2 wk or 0.05% daily rinse reduces caries by 40 %.
- Systemic F ingestion is more selective in decreasing caries on smooth surface than P and F surfaces.
- P and F sealants = reapplication after 6 mos.

Preventive resin restorations = PRR are of 3 types, i.e.

1. Type A = suspicious P and F where caries removal is limited to enamel.
2. Type B = incipient lesions in dentin which is small and confined.
3. Type C = i.e. greater exploration of dentin is required.

TREATMENT of F^- toxicity –

S. no.	Levels; mg / kg body wt	Treatments
1	< 5.0	Milk/Ca^{++};
2	5 – 15	Ca^{++}; induce vomiting; gastric lavage
3	> 15	Induce vomiting; cardiac monitoring; I/V 10 ml of 10 % of Ca gluconate; hospitalise; diuretics for increasing urine output

TOPICAL FLUORIDES

2 % NaF

- Was the **first topically applied F compound.**
- 2 %; 4 applications = 40 % reduction in caries occurs.
- 20 gm of NaF powder in 1000 ml of water.
- 3 – 4 min is the application time.
- At 3, 7, 11, 13 yrs of age which coincides with the eruption of new teeth. It is ka **Knutson's technique**.
- 4 applications are done at an interval of 1 week difference (4 visits × 4 times in a year) × 4 times in life so a **total 64 applications** are required – is its disadvantages also.
- No pigmentations of teeth occurs.

8% SnF_2 = given by **Muhler**

- Enamel is more acid resistant as compared to NaF, etc.
- **Annual application** / single regimen.
- Fresh solutions should be prepared for each patient, because it is unstable.
- Applied for 4 min on the teeth.
- 30 – 40 % caries reductions.
- But causes pigmentation and staining of teeth.

1.23 % APF = aka **Brudevold's solution**

1. Currently, it is **the most widely used solution.**
2. Causes increased uptake of F by enamel as cp with NaF / SnF2.
3. 70 % decreased DMF surfaces.
4. APF contains **NaF as active ingredient**. The formula has 1.23 % of F as NaF buffered to a pH of 3 – 4 in a 0.1 M phosphoric acid.
5. 20 gm of NaF in 1 liter of 0.1 M phosphoric acid + 50 % HF (for pH = 3) gives F ions 1.23 %.
6. APF gel **pH = 4 – 5**
7. Applied at 6 or 12 mos. Interval.
8. Application time = 4 min.
9. Main advantage = is its **ability to deposit F in enamel to a deeper depth** than NaF / SnF_2.

10. But it should not be stored in glass containers because HF has etching properties.

VARNISHES

- Duraphet = caries rate decreases by 30 – 40 % in permanent teeth. It contains 5 % NaF, i.e. 2.26 % F.
- Fluorprotector = is difluorosilane; silane fluoride with 0.7 % of F = 7000 ppm F.
- Carex = 1.8 % F;
- Varnishes are better than other topical F agents in depositing F in sound enamel.
- 0.3 – 0.5 ml varnish for full dentition applied for 4 min.

Mechanism of action

1. Ca^{++} in HA + NaF = ➔ CaF_2 — + HA ➔ HFA
2. HA + SnF_2 ➔ stannous trifluorophosphate, which is more resistant to decay; + HFA + **metallic taste** is due to tin hydroxy phosphate.
3. APF = it causes **shrinkage of the volume of HA crystals** due to dehydration and so F can penetrate more deeply through these openings in enamel to form HFA.
4. Acidification of F solution with phosphoric acid provides a low pH, favouring F deposition.
5. Amine F, i.e. organic fluoride compounds; better than the SnF_2, APF, because it provides **amine portion** which has **both surfactants and antimicrobial properties.**

FLUORIDATED DENTIFRICES = give 0.1 % F mainly.

1. NaF = 0.24 % NaF ; gives 0.11 % F; **do not stain the teeth;** dentifrices should not have the $CaCO_3$, i.e. Ca – containing compounds which will otherwise react with F to form CaF_2.
2. SnF_2 = Muhler 1956 found 8 % SnF_2 topical and 0.4 % SnF_2 in dentifrices. But it **causes staining of teeth**, pigmentation of restorative margins; metallic taste in mouth.
3. Na – MFP = 0.7 % which gives 0.1 % F = it reduces 17 – 34 % caries.
4. Amine fluorides = give F 0.125 %.

Dental caries

Enamel caries = earliest clinical appearance of caries is a **white spot**, caused by the loss of Ca and phosphate ions from the enamel **prisms. Initial loss is subsurface only**. May become discolored ka brown spot lesion.

Occult caries = is the **extensive dentin caries** in the p.o. minimal or no clinically apparent enamel breakdown. Most commonly occurs under occlusal surfaces.

Recurrent caries = continuation of caries after placement of the restoration.

Secondary caries = new caries occurring at restoration margins.

Rampant caries = i.e. gross caries in deciduous dentition, involving those areas of tooth not susceptible to causes.

Nursing bottle caries = i.e. extensive caries in primary incisors due to prolonged exposure to sugar containing drinks in bottle feeding; esp. involves maxillary anteriors; mandibular anteriors escape due to saliva and tongue coverage.

Caries can be difficult to diagnose by clinical examination alone, so bitewing r/g should be taken if required.

Fibre optic transillumination FOTI = a bright light is conducted along fibre optic cable and is directed in I/D areas, the caries appears as a dark shadow.

Dyes = used for cavity preparation; dye is taken by the carious dentin.

DMFT index = i.e. decayed, missing, filled index is the most widely used method of recording the caries experience.

DMFT = applies to the permanent teeth.

DMFS = applies to permanent tooth surfaces.

dmft/dmfs applies to the deciduous teeth.

Components of DMF can be used to determine —

1. Index of Rx need = D / DMF
2. Index of restorative provision **aka care index** = F / DMF
3. Index of Rx failure = M / DMF

OTHER IMPORTANT POINTS

- 2% NaF was used in first artificial water fluoridation
- Unstimulated saliva contains a higher F^- conc. than stimulated saliva.
- Saliva/plasma ratio is about 0.6 at the maximum dose.
- Plasma F^- increases with age over the range of 10–38 years.
- If water is having less than 0.25 ppm F^-, the mean conc of F^- in blood is about 0.5 μmol/l (0.01 ppm).

Model Test Paper

Orthodontics

1. **Crossbites are often seen in the developing dentition in the molar region. Treatment should always be as follows;**
   A. Both molars should be moved equal amounts for correction
   B. One molar should be moved the entire distance for correction
   C. The possibility of functional interference and shift of the mandible should be considered.
   D. One molar should be extracted.

2. **There is a differential between girls and boys with respect to the age at which the growth velocity reaches its peak. That difference is;**
   A. Boys six months ahead of girls
   B. Girls six months ahead of boys
   C. Girls one year ahead of boys
   D. Girls two years ahead of boys

3. **The major etiologic factor responsible for Class II malocclusion is;**
   A. Sleeping habits
   B. Growth discrepancy
   C. Thumb and tongue habits
   D. Tooth to jaw size discrepancy

4. **In cephalometric analysis of children with malocclusion, the angle ANB is frequently used. In patients with severe Class II malocclusion this angle is;**
   A. Large
   B. Small
   C. Normal
   D. Negative

5. A ten-year old patient has mandibular canines trying to erupt into a space insufficient by 2 mm. Primary second molars are large and firmly in place. First premolars are erupting. An acceptable preventive orthodontic procedure for this case would be:

A. Disking the mesial proximals of the mandibular primary second molars.
B. Extracting the mandibular primary second molars.
C. Placing a removable bite opener
D. Extracting the first premolars

6. Most Class II malocclusions can be prevented by;

A. Maintaining the integrity of the primary dentition
B. Preventing deleterious habits such as thumb sucking, lip biting, etc.
C. Breast feeding
D. No known technique
E. (1), (2) and (3) above

7. In a mixed dentition space analysis, the most careful estimate will only be accurate within

A. 0.5 mm
B. 2.0 mm
C. 4.0 mm
D. 6.0 mm

8. The purpose of employing loops and helices in wires in tooth moving appliances is to

A. Provide a lighter force
B. Provide a longer lever arm
C. Lengthen the period between adjustment
D. All of the above

9. In correcting an anterior cross bite, the appliance to be used is determined by the;

A. Amount of overbite
B. Age of the patient
C. Cooperation of the patient
D. All of the above

10. At birth, which of the following structures is nearest the size it will eventually attain in adulthood?

A. Cranium
B. Mandible
C. Clavicle
D. Middle face
E. Nasal capsule

11. A 13-year child has a 3 mm maxillary midline diastema and a heavy fibrous midline frenum. The child exhibits an otherwise normal occlusion. Which of the following is the best approach to managing this problem?

A. Band the central incisors and use a space closing device and then excise the frenum.
B. Band the central incisors and close the space with extra oral force
C. Excise the tissue between the central incisor and close the diastema orthodontically
D. Excise the tissue between the central incisors and permit the diastema to close on its own.

12. A malocclusion is characterized by contraction of the maxillary denture, labioversion of maxillary incisors, deep overbite and overjet. These are typical characteristics of a malocclusion of which of the following Angle classification?

A. Class I
B. Class II, Division 1
C. Class II, Division 2
D. Class III

13. The optimal time to employ an orthodontic appliance that takes advantage of growth is during;

A. Late primary dentition
B. Early mixed dentition
C. Late mixed dentition
D. Early permanent dentition

14. The band and crib space maintainer is classified as;

A. Bilateral, fixed and functional
B. Unilateral, fixed and functional

C. Unilateral, fixed and nonfunctional
D. Unilateral, removable and nonfunctional

15. The "V" principle of growth is best illustrated by the;
A. Nasal septum
B. Mandibular ramus
C. Mandibular symphysis
D. Spheno-occipital synchondrosis

Local anaesthesia

16. A patient develops a typical Bell's palsy facial expression within 10 minutes after an attempted inferior alveolar nerve block on the same side. The most logical explanation is that the injection was into the;
A. Parotid gland
B. Maxillary artery
C. Buccinator muscle
D. Temporalis muscle
E. Pterygomandibular ligament

17. Trismus following inferior alveolar nerve block most likely results from;
A. Failure to use an aspirating syringe
B. Irritation of the medial pterygoid muscle
C. Accidental injection of the solution near a branch of the facial nerve
D. Allowing the needle tip to rest beneath the periosteum during injection
E. Accidental injection of the solution near a major motor branch of the trigeminal nerve

18. Which of the following mandibular teeth may be removed without pain after administration of an inferior alveolar and lingual nerve block?
A. All molars
B. Canine and first premolar
C. All teeth in the quadrant
D. Both premolars and first molar

19. Which of the following muscles is most frequently encountered in an incorrect anterior superior alveolar (infraorbital) nerve block?

A. Mentalis
B. Risorius
C. Triangularis
D. Orbicularis oris
E. Quadratus labii-superioris

20. An edentulous patient requires removal of the mylohyoid ridge. Which of the following nerves should be protected?

A. Lingual
B. Mental
C. Mylohyoid
D. Inferior alveolar

21. Instead of responding to treatment for syncope, the patient's pulse and respiration become weak and irregular with attendant cyanosis. The first resuscitative measure should be to;

A. Begin closed chest cardiac massage
B. Inject 40 mg of Wyamine®
C. Support circulation by injection 1:1,000 epinephrine
D. Raise the blood CO_2 by placing a paper bag over the patient's face.
E. Support respiration with oxygen through an open airway

22. How many milligrams of epinephrine are in each cartridge (1.8 cc) of 2 per cent lidocaine with 1:100000 (epinephrine)

A. 0.018 mg
B. 0.036 mg
C. 0.18 mg
D. 0.36 mg
E. 3.6 mg

23. A 40-lbs. child required multiple dental procedures under local anesthesia. The maximum number of cartridges of lidocaine with 1:100000 epinephrine that may be safely administered at one time is;

A. 1
B. 3

C. 5
D. 8
E. 10

24. A 19-year old patient requires extraction of all erupted teeth because of extensive decay. If the patient has two maxillary third molars that are full bony impactions, the molars should be;
A. Retained, as they will never erupt
B. Extracted along with other teeth
C. Surgically exposed and possibly used for prosthetic retention
D. Retained under a denture until they erupt

25. Three days after full mouth extraction an elderly patient complains the "black and blue marks on her neck". The most probable diagnosis is;
A. Leukemia
B. Polycythemia
C. Thrombocytopenia
D. Postoperative ecchymosis

26. Most reactions following injection of local anesthetic agents are caused by;
A. Anxiety
B. Toxicity
C. Allergies
D. Overdosage
E. Intraarterial injections

27. Hematoma formation during or immediately following a posterior superior alveolar block anesthesia is most likely a result of damage to the;
A. Facial artery
B. Pterygoid venous plexus
C. Internal maxillary artery
D. Small capillaries and the arterioles

28. Two minutes following cessation of a two-hour treatment session using 80 per cent nitrous oxide, 20 per cent oxygen

and local anesthesia, the patient becomes cyanotic and tachycardiac. The most probable explanation is;

A. Over-oxygenation
B. Under-oxygenation
C. Diffusion hypoxia
D. Malignant hyperthermia

29. Treatment of syncope is most effectively accomplished by;

A. Calling a physician
B. Administering 100 percent oxygen for five minutes
C. Lowering the chair to place the patient's head lower than his feet and massaging his face and neck with a cold, wet towel.
D. Bending the patient's head forward between his knees and asking the patient to raise his head against hand pressure

Oral Pathology and Dental Radiology

30. An oral condition which predisposes an individual to an increase in the incidence and rate of development of dental caries is;

A. Xerostomia
B. Leukoplakia
C. Pharyngitis
D. Herpes stomatitis
E. Median rhomboid glossitis

31. The most common malignancy within the oral cavity is the;

A. Ameloblastoma
B. Adenocarcinoma
C. Basal cell carcinoma
D. Malignant mixed tumor
E. Squamous cell carcinoma

32. The characteristic lesion of herpes virus infections on the skin or mucous membranes is;

A. Necrosis
B. Tunnel action
C. Hyperketatosis
D. Abscess
E. Vesicle

33. A maxillary lateral incisor with non vital pulp and with periapical radiolucency is suitably treated and the root canal appropriately obturated after two successive negative cultures of the apical area. The most common result of such treatment is;

A. Radiographic resolution of the periapical lesion within 2-3 weeks and an uneventful subsequent history
B. Radiographic resolution of the periapical lesion within 6-12 months and an uneventful subsequent history
C. No change at the periapical area during 12 months or more, subsequent history otherwise uneventful.
D. Reappearance within 12 months of symptoms attributable to periapical infection.

34. Two or more teeth united only by cementum is designated as;

A. Fusion
B. Sclerosis
C. Gemination
D. Dilaceration
E. Concrescence

35. In normal dental diagnostic procedures, the principal radiation hazard to the operator is produced by;

A. Gamma radiation
B. Primary radiation
C. Secondary radiation
D. None of the above

36. The radiopacity that frequently obliterates the apices of maxillary molars when using the bisecting principle of the intraoral radiography is the;

A. Zygoma and the zygomatic process of the maxilla
B. Orbital process of the zygomatic bone
C. Palatine bone and the zygoma
D. Maxillary sinus

37. "Sulfur granules" are of diagnostic value in suspected cases of;

A. Actinomycosis
B. Blastomycosis

C. Syphilis
D. Hensen's disease
E. Candidiasis

38. A young woman is admitted to the hospital. Petechiae on the oral mucous membrane and marginal gingival hemorrhage are noted. Platelet count is 15,000 /mm^3 with increases in bleeding and clot retraction time. The RBC and differential are normal. Probable diagnosis is;
A. Infectious mononucleosis
B. Thrombocytopenic purpura
C. Monocytic leukemia
D. Pernicious anemia
E. Hemophilia

39. Characteristic dental findings of cleidocranial dysostosis include;
A. Increased caries susceptibility
B. Enamel hypoplasia and lack of enamel formation
C. Juvenile periodontosis and subsequent premature loss of death
D. Failure of shedding and eruption, and numerous unerupted supernumerary teeth
E. All of the above

40. Multiple giant cell lesions of bone are associated with;
A. Pituitary deficiency
B. Hyperparathyroidism
C. Addison's disease
D. Hypothyroidism
E. Diabetes

41. The rarefaction occurring in the bone from an infected deciduous molar, as studied radiographically, most frequently appears;
A. About the apices
B. Between two teeth
C. In the bifurcation
D. Around the developing permanent tooth
E. As a uniform widening of the periodontal ligament space

42. A congenital epulis of the new born is most likely to resemble microscopically

A. An epithelial pearl
B. A gingivitis granuloma gravidarium
C. An aberrant sebaceous gland
D. A granular cell myoblastoma
E. A peripheral giant cell granuloma

43. The radiographic examination of a patient 20-year old disclosed a circumscribed radiolucent lesion 2 cm in diameter in the mandibular right molar region. The lesion was sharply outlined but lacked a radiopaque periphery, was somewhat irregularly shaped and extended 5 to 6 mm above the apices of the molars and 10 mm inferiorly towards the lower border of the mandible. There was no evidence of the bone and the lesion was asymptomatic. All teeth tested within a normal vitality range. These findings would suggest;

A. Dentigerous cyst
B. Radicular cyst
C. Compound odontoma
D. Simple bone cyst

44. Caries on a proximal surface usually starts;

A. Buccal to the contact zone and the marginal ridge
B. Lingual to the contract zone and the marginal ridge
C. Between the contact zone and the dentinoenamel junction
D. Between the contact zone and the crest of the gingiva
E. Distal to the contact zone
F. At the contact zone

45. An inflamed capillary hemangioma of the oral cavity looks similar, microscopically, to

A. A nevus
B. A neurofibroma
C. An angiosarcoma
D. A pyogenic granuloma

46. A periapical radiograph of the mandibular premolar region reveals a completely embedded supernumerary tooth, superimposed on the roots of both premolars. With another

film in the same position a second projection is made from a more mesial horizontal angulation. In the second film, the image of the supernumerary tooth, appears to have shifted distally from its original position. This would indicate that the supernumerary tooth lies;

A. Buccal to the premolars
B. Lingual to the premolars
C. In the same plane as the premolars

47. A patient complains of numbness of the lower lip. There is no history of tooth extraction. The condition is likely to be related to;

A. Infection
B. Metastatic neoplasm
C. Dental manipulation
D. Disease of the central nervous system

48. Ground sections of early dental caries of enamel exhibit;

A. Accentuated bands of Retzius and cross striations of enamel rods.
B. Zones of fatty degeneration and sclerosis of enamel rods.
C. Accentuated Owen's lines of contour and marked interglobular areas
D. Zones of fatty degeneration and interglobular enamel

49. A junction of roots of adjacent teeth through cemental union is termed;

A. Fusion
B. Gemination
C. Concrescence
D. Megalodontia
E. Dilacceration

50. A major radiographic finding is ectodermal dysplasia is;

A. A ground-glass appearance of the bone.
B. Many congenitally missing teeth
C. Calcification of the falx of cerebrum
D. Hutchinson's teeth
E. Osteoporosis

51. A unilateral progressive decrease in the size of the facial tissues resulting from a neurovascular abnormality is known as;

A. Ankylosis
B. Hemiatrophy
C. Hemihypertrophy
D. Leontiasis ossea

52. Pleomorphic adenomas of parotid gland origin are most likely to exhibit;

A. Rapid growth with early death of the patient.
B. Early metastasis to distant organs
C. Slow growth but a tendency to local recurrence after incomplete removal.
D. Latent metastasis after local removal.
E. Early ulceration and hemorrhage

53. A patient has a swelling of long standing at the ala of the nose on the left side. Examination reveals a swelling in the floor of the nostril and beneath the upper lip. There is no pain and regional teeth are vital. Radiographs show no bone change. The preliminary diagnosis would be;

A. Alveolar abscess
B. Incisive canal cyst
C. Nasolabial cyst
D. Dermoid cyst
E. Maxillary sinusitis

54. Some microorganisms produce a diffuse spreading, inflammatory reaction due to the elaboration of;

A. Coagulase
B. Peroxidase
C. Bradykinin
D. Hyaluronidase

55. Intraoral radiographic examination of a 40-year old woman disclosed a series of circumscribed periapical radiolucent

lesions with areas of radiopacity within them involving the six mandibular anterior teeth. Every tooth was vital, normal in colour and asymptomatic. These findings suggest;

A. Cementomas
B. Osteomalacia
C. Simple bone cysts
D. Condensing osteitis

Answer Key to MCQs in Model Text Paper

1	C	2	D	3	B	4	A
5	A	6	B	7	A	8	A
9	D	10	A	11	A	12	B
13	C	14	C	15	B	16	A
17	B	18	D	19	E	20	A
21	E	22	A	23	B	24	D
25	D	26	A	27	B	28	C
29	C	30	A	31	E	32	E
33	B	34	E	35	C	36	A
37	A	38	B	39	D	40	B
41	C	42	E	43	D	44	C
45	D	46	A	47	B	48	A
49	C	50	B	51	B	52	C
53	C	54	D	55	A		

Appendix

TABLE I

1.	Maximum growth of skull completed by	6–7 years
2.	Most cranial sutures close by	5 years
3.	Cranial vault attains size nearest the size of adulthood	at Birth
4.	Maximum inter canine width in mandible is completed by	9–10 years
5.	Mid-symphyseal suture fuses at age	$\underline{\propto}$ 18 mos ($\underline{\propto}$ 2 years age)
6.	Spheno-occipital synchondrosis closes at	18–25 years
7.	Growth of Anterior cranial base completed by	6–7 years
8.	CP occurs in	8–10 week IU
9.	Inter canine width in maxilla completed by	10–12 years
10.	Maxillary sinus is first to develop and starts developing at	4 months IU
11.	Papillae of tongue are seen by	11 week IU
12.	Taste buds in circumvallate papillae	12 week IU
13.	Taste buds in fungi form papillae	14 week IU
14.	Metopic suture of skull fuses by	5th year
15.	Anterior and posterior fontanelles close by	1st yr age
16.	cleft lip and jaw would be apparent by	6th–7th week IU
17.	Developmental malformations of face occur during	4–12 week IU
18.	Union of palatine processes is completed by	3 month IU
19.	Greatest period of cranial growth	0–5 years
20.	Vestibule (oral) is apparent by	6 week IU

21.	Buccopharyngeal membrane persists upto	4 week IU
22.	Oronasal membrane ruptures at	6 week IU
23.	Nasobuccal membrane ruptures at	5 week IU
24.	Palate formation starts at and goes upto	5–12 week IU
25.	Thyroglossal duct disappears by	7 week IU
26.	Primary and secondary ossification centres appear at	6th week & 9 months IU
27.	Pharyngeal arches develop by	4th week IU
28.	All PNS grow rapidly at	6–7 year of age
29.	Mid palatal suture does not close until	6–7 year of age
30.	Increase in width of maxilla is mostly completed by	10–12 year of age

TABLE II

1.	Time of initiation of permanent first molar is (Bud develops)	4 mo IU
2.	Calcification of first permanent molars starts at	Birth
3.	At what age = 12 primary + 12 permanent erupted teeth	8.5 years
4.	First evidence of calcification of IInd premolars	1½–2½ years
5.	Teeth initiated after birth	4, 5, 7, 8
6.	Jaws of newborn child show calcification of	24 teeth
7.	Enamel of permanent incisors forms between	Birth–5 years age
8.	Enamel formation/ crown formation of all primary teeth completed by	1–11 months
9.	Time required for primary teeth to reach occlusion after cutting into oral cavity is	2–12 months
10.	Initiation of primary tooth bud is (first bud)	6 week IU

11.	First evidence of calcification of primary. teeth	4 months IU (17 week IU)
12.	Crowns of all permanent teeth except M3 complete by	8 years
13.	Permanent tooth takes _____ years to complete apex closure after eruption	2½–3 years
14.	Enamel formation occurs between	4 month IU to 12–16 years
15.	Bud of M2 starts at	1 year age
16.	Bud of M3 starts at	4–5 year age

MISCELLANEOUS

⇒ Head begins to take shape = 21 day

⇒ Oral plate ruptures = 4th week

⇒ Primordia for facial development are readily seen = at 5th week IU

⇒ Branchial arches, pharyngeal pouches = 5th week

⇒ Centres of endochondral ossifications appear leaving only the synchondroses = 7th week

⇒ **Dental development starts = 3rd mo. IUL life M**

⇒ Tongue is formed from 1, 3, 4th branchial arches

⇒ Taste buds = 2nd arch = 7th N

⇒ Early MDP = 612 eruption upto 6–8 years

⇒ Late MDP = 345 eruption 10–12 years

⇒ 2½ years = all primary teeth (present) erupted.

⇒ 3 years = roots of all deciduous teeth complete, crowns of permanent first molars complete, roots start developing.

⇒ 9–10 years age = all permanent teeth except M3 have completed crown formation and enamel deposition.

⇒ Teeth usually erupt when 3/4th of their roots are completed.

⇒ 2–3 years are required for roots to be completed after tooth has come in occlusion.

⇒ Roots of all incisors and M 1 completed by = Dental age 11 (eleven)

⇒ Roots of all permanent teeth (upto M2) completed by = Dental age 15.

⇒ Teeth erupt 5 mos earlier in F than M2.

Palatal shelves unite by 8½ week IU

⇒ Mid-palatal suture ossifies by 12–14 years.

Reader's Notes

Reader's Notes

Reader's Notes

Reader's Notes